I Love

But... I Love Me More!

Banish Metabolic Syndrome, the Gateway to Chronic Disease, for a Longer, Sexier Life

By Mary Kay Matossian

BSN, Biometrics Wellness Nurse

Illustrations by

Leslie Hinton

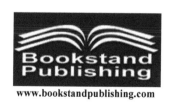

www.bookstandpublishing.com

Published by
Bookstand Publishing
Pasadena, CA 91101
4824_3

ISBN 978-1-953710-06-2

Disclaimer

No part of this publication may be reproduced or transmitted in any form or by any means, mechanical or electronic, including photocopying or recording, or by any information storage and retrieval system, or transmitted by email without permission in writing from the author. Neither the author nor the publisher assumes any responsibility for errors, omissions, or contrary interpretations of the subject matter herein. Any perceived slight of any individual or organization is purely unintentional.

Brand and product names are trademarks or registered trademarks of their respective owners.

This book is meant to delight, surprise and inspire you. In no way is this book offering medical advice. The information is educational and entertaining. Upon using any information contained in this book, you agree to hold the author harmless against any damages, costs, and expenses, including any legal fees, potentially resulting from the application of any information provided by this book. This disclaimer applies to any damages caused by the use and application, whether directly or indirectly, of any advice or information presented, or under any other cause of action.

You agree to accept all risks of using the information presented in this book.

The fact that several individuals, organizations, and such related documents, referenced in this book, does not imply that the author or publisher endorses the information that the individual or organization provided. This is an unofficial analytical review of much of the data related to the whole-food, plant-based diet, and lifestyle. This book has not been approved by the original sources and institutions that discovered the science behind a whole-food, plant-based diet.

Mary Kay Matossian
the.blood.challenge@gmail.com
www.thebloodchallenge.com

"I warn you: if you read this book, you will never quite think about food the same way again. You will never quite think about your body the same way. You will never quite think about your health the same way. And, you will never quite think about your life the same way. It's not that Mary Matossian tells you things you might not have heard or read before; it's that she puts things together in a way that makes healthier eating seem more understandable, and more attainable. This book is not only informative, it's inspiring and motivating. It's a real gift to those who are seeking a healthier body and a happier, clearer mind."

**Marianne Williamson,
New York Best Selling Author**

For my husband,
Harry Berj Matossian,
physician and gastroenterologist:

The precious man who never gives up.
Thank you for believing…

"Truth is not what I believe. Truth is fact. I may not believe it. I may not know it. That does not change it. It is there nevertheless, waiting to be discovered and believed. Truth does not depend on the unsettled and changing opinions of men. It was truth before it was believed. It will remain truth whether it is believed or not."

Carlyle B. Haynes

Table of Contents

1. What's Wrong with Me?

D o you ever ask yourself, "Where did all my energy go?" Once, you were full of hope and aspirations. Now, you are barely there, tired and gaining weight fast! How did you arrive at this disappointing place in life, and you are so young? You gain weight easily; and, no matter what you do or do not do, the weight keeps creeping on. You feel robbed, and deliberately misguided. Your future is not so bright as you battle brain fog, fatigue, and constant disappointment. You feel hoodwinked, misguided, and undermined by your diminishing health and a lack of energy and mental prowess. You follow all the *rules*, but you are confused, depressed, and angry. Health magazines, science, and research studies from reputable institutions constantly conflict with one another. One corporation tells you to eat one thing, and another corporation or scientific study tells you to eat something completely different! It's not fair! You don't know who to believe, and you are confused! Confusion causes paralysis. You don't know the rules, so you do nothing. An evolutionary biologist E.O. Wilson states:

"We're drowning in a sea of information while starving for wisdom."

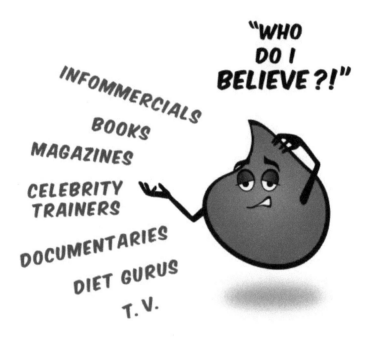

You work hard for every dollar you make, and you wonder, "How will I pay for my health bills?" Your diminishing health, doctor visits and treatments take up valuable time and resources. Every doctor visit leads to more doctor visits with added prescriptions and procedures. You are amidst a slow, cruel, and impoverishing demise that cannot be stopped, except when you take more prescriptions!

You are a typical American patient walking into a primary care provider's office. Your physician will announce you are obese with a Body Mass Index (BMI) of 30. Your blood pressure will be 150/105, and you will be diagnosed with hypertension. Antihypertensive medications such as lisinopril and/or metoprolol will be prescribed. Your basic bloodwork will show a fasting blood glucose of 140 and a hemoglobin A1C of 7. You have a new diagnosis of type 2 diabetes, and you begin your insulin medication, metformin and/or glipizide. Your fasting cholesterol will be 250, and your triglycerides above 300. You start Lipitor because you have hyperlipidemia, which is too much fat circulating in your blood. Your doctor tells you about the dangerous side effects of Lipitor, *but* does not tell you about the dangerous side effects of your food choices which contribute to all of your diagnoses! Your doctor tells you:

You have Metabolic Syndrome,
High Blood Pressure,
High Blood Glucose, and
High Cholesterol.

At this point, you are confused and alarmed. Friends and family are giving you advice, but everyone's advice is conflicting! You complain about daytime sleepiness and fatigue, and you have a history of snoring and erratic breathing at night with loud noises. You wake up often from the sound of your own snoring, and feel tired in the morning. Another diagnosis is added: obstructive sleep apnea. You are prescribed a C-PAP machine to improve your breathing throughout the night. Because of your weight gain, you experience pain in your neck, back, hips, and knees. Your feet have a burning sensation on a regular basis, including first thing in the morning. You take prescription pain pills and sleeping pills which have dangerous side effects. The human skeleton is not designed to carry an extra 60 to 150 or more pounds. The added wear and tear on the spine and big joints cause arthritis pain. Therefore, you are prescribed Celebrex and/or a stronger pain medication called Tramadol. Due to all these conditions, you complain of anxiety, depression, and workplace dysfunction. Cymbalta, BuSpar, and Elavil are also prescribed to help you deal with these new diagnoses. You're trapped.

What frustrates you the most about your dilemma is that everyone tells you, "This is normal aging." You manage work commitments, computers, emails, staff issues, coworkers, kids' schedules, and finances, but you cannot manage your own body and disgruntled moods. What are the rules for having great health? You are winning at business, family, multi-tasking, and capitalism, but you have lost the ultimate goal: A healthy body and mind. You know something is wrong, but you cannot figure it out! You have a manual on how to conquer all aspects of your life, but how to take care of your body is a mystery.

You say "No" to new opportunities and invitations because you are tired, out of breath, out of shape, out of time, and overwhelmed. You cannot add another thing to your schedule, even if it is pleasant. You keep seeing a vision of your future self: A youthful, carefree senior who is full of vitality, strength, curiosity, and intelligence, who enjoys others and never misses a beat! You do not want to be younger; you just want to feel great and grow old on your own terms! The vision of your future self is going away. These chronic ailments rob you of precious time and prevent you from exercising, going on adventures, meeting new people, and completing work assignments in a prompt fashion because of brain fog, fatigue, and chronic malaise. Most weekends, you are finishing up last week's assignments and catching up on everyday tasks. Consequently, you postpone precious time with your kids, loved ones, and recreational activities. You cannot work any harder! If you do not change your energy level now, you will continue this downward spiral of misery leading to death. As E.O. Wilson said:

"We must think and live differently
NOW
if we are going to survive."

For no obvious reason, you cannot sleep at night, and reality hits you. When you awaken at night, your heart races so fast you gasp for air and remind yourself, "Everything is okay…Right?" You wonder if this is all in your head. Fear, grief, and despair overwhelm you. It feels like you are being punished. You are smart, caring, and doing your best, but quality of life eludes you. Where does all this fear come from? You have tried everything. Losing weight is impossible. You eat so little, and it leaves you more tired, irritable, deprived, and hungry.

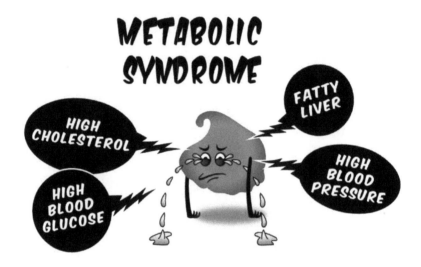

You have metabolic syndrome: high blood pressure, high cholesterol, high blood glucose levels, and a fatty liver. You are in a losing battle, and it is expensive. You must do something about this problem, now! Each year will get worse. Many adults already have diabetes, which impacts all aspects of health and mortality. You are all too familiar with diminishing dreams as you observe the downward spiral of your aging parents and the cost of keeping them out of the hospital. How do you get rid of these aches, pains, anxiety, and prescription drugs? You don't know what to do. However, the solution is hidden in plain sight...

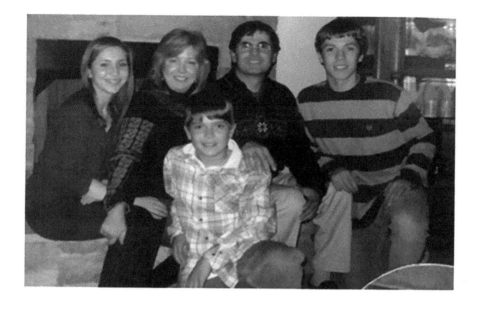

What Is Metabolic Syndrome?

Metabolic syndrome is chronic, constant inflammation which is the gateway to chronic disease. Its main cause is the Standard American Diet (or SAD), which is high in animal cholesterol, containing extra hormones, and fat which our bodies do not need. This animal cholesterol doesn't know where to go, and so it collects in our arteries, muscles and surrounding fat. Animal cholesterol interferes with microcirculation. As arteries get stiff and narrow, your blood pressure begins to rise. Excess cholesterol blocks insulin from getting glucose into cells for energy. This is microcirculation. Animal cholesterol gets in the way of everything! It is an unwanted "house guest" who will not leave! Animal cholesterol blocks tiny blood vessels nourishing our heart, liver, eyes, pancreas, and brain. Animal cholesterol converts to plaque within blood vessels

7

and fat storage throughout the body. Metabolic syndrome is *not* an isolated medical condition. It is a systemic inflammatory, microcirculation problem that impacts your health in every way...

What is the cost to have a body and mind full of energy, strength, joy, compassion and focus?

What is the cost to have an unhealthy body and foggy mind during these tumultuous times? What is the personal cost of needless suffering and endless frustrations? You are smart; why can't you figure this out? What information do you believe, and why? Did you agree to a shorter, miserable lifespan riddled with ailments? ***You deserve better***! Now is the time to say *no* to needless suffering and financial loss. A life free from chronic disease, inflammation, brain fog, fatigue, despair, and weight gain *is* a powerful elixir worth exploring... It's closer than you think. Simple changes create enormous improvements that energize your body and mind to thrive in challenging times.

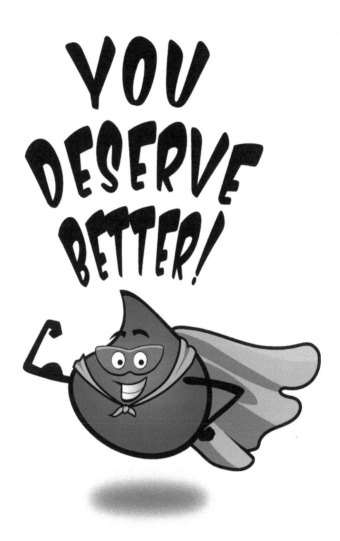

Mary Kay Matossian

2. I'm a Biometrics RN: I Can Help!

I don't know about you, but I ***LOVE*** bacon and eggs! A high-protein diet makes so much sense, right? In the past, each of my meals had chicken, salmon, and beef. Eating right is important. I followed all the recommended diet and food trends from highly regarded sources. I believed in a high-protein diet, and I was getting results. There is so much at stake taking care of our bodies and minds because so much is expected of us! I wanted to do what's right for my family and me, but my health and wellness didn't match up to all my efforts! Why did I feel so lousy?

After twelve years of suffering from metabolic syndrome, I am shocked by the simple cure. Metabolic syndrome *is* the gateway to inflammatory, chronic diseases including diabetes, autoimmune disorders, stroke, heart attack, mental illness, dementia, Alzheimer's, and early death. As a nurse in the healthcare industry for twenty-five years, how did I miss this information? I took continuing education classes online, around the country, and all over the world. As an informed healthcare provider and administrator, I was keeping up with science. So how did I miss these data?

I will never forget when at age 45 I was first diagnosed with metabolic syndrome. I asked my wise, experienced internal medicine physician, "What's metabolic syndrome?"

His sheepish response: "These are the symptoms of being fat. Your vital organs are surrounded by a dangerous fat that's harming your health."

At that point, I could not consume any fewer calories than I already was because my metabolism had come to a grinding halt! If I looked at a split pea, I would gain weight! Metabolic syndrome is high blood pressure, high cholesterol, high blood glucose, and abdominal obesity. After all these years, I finally had a real diagnosis, and I felt defeated. How on earth do you lose weight with metabolic syndrome? I became depressed, and I realized I was in trouble.

My Lifespan is shortening…

I chose to fight for a better life, no matter what that would look like or cost me. I began by studying the ancient spiritual principles of yoga and how yogic body postures represent spiritual truths. Yoga has been around for 24,000 years and is still flourishing! Maybe there's something to it? I took the time to study, practice, and memorize Sanskrit words and yogic postures.

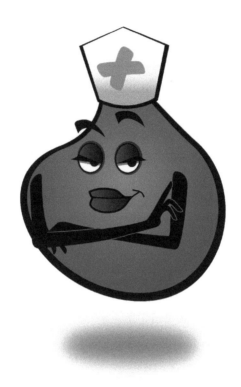

Then, I studied meditation and how it connects our heart, soul, and body. Relationships, focused on core values and service, create joy and happiness. I am getting somewhere! Meditation became a part of my daily life. I continued to ask the question, "Why am I here?"

On two separate trips to India, I studied and practiced Ayurvedic Medicine, yoga, and meditation. Each time, I was "miraculously healed" from metabolic syndrome… for a little while. But I couldn't go to India every time I felt lousy. Within a few weeks of returning from each of my trips to India, I became ill again: Anxious, bloated, angry, and gaining weight. My blood pressure, glucose, and cholesterol rose to dangerous levels! What was the connection? What was making me healthy in India, but deathly ill in the United States? Was it the intense heat, fasting, and/or the humidity? Was it the yoga, meditation, community, or swimming in the Arabic Sea? What was working each time I traveled to India? I did not make the connection.

At this point in my life, I was willing to do anything for reasonable health! As a final effort, I went to the famous True North Clinic in Santa Rosa, California, which specializes in water-fasting and a whole-food plant-based diet, free of salt, oil, and sugar. Exasperated and out of hope, I thought, "I'll give it a four-day trial!" At the True North Clinic, I ate three plant-based meals per day without salt, sugar, and oil until I was full.

Whole Food, Plant-based (***WFPB***) meals consist of boiled and raw vegetables, grains, beans/legumes, fruits, nuts, oatmeal, and dried fruits such as raisins. Herbs, fresh lemon and non-spicy condiments were available for my salad and seasoning my food. Throughout the day and between meals, I drank water and herbal teas. This was the same as I had done in India! What could this short, four-day stay possibly do for me?

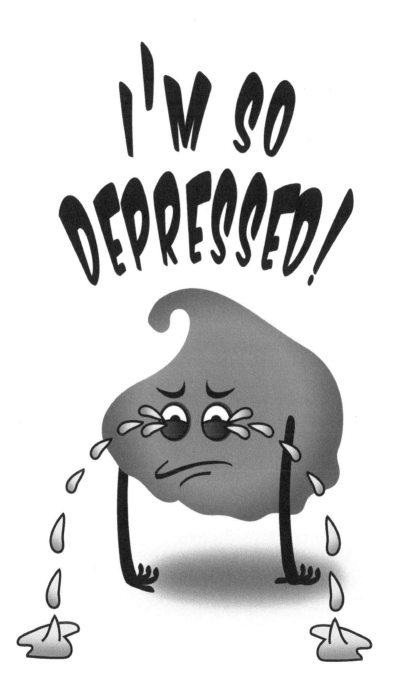

The answer is this: After four days, my systolic blood pressure dropped a staggering 60 points, from 170/110 to 110/70, and I lost seven pounds of water weight! For another 90 days, I continued on the **WFPB** diet, which is whole grains, beans, vegetables and fruit. My total cholesterol went from 240 to 130 mg/dL. This experience was shocking. A simple food change radically changed my life. After a few months, my cholesterol blood levels were so low, my homeopathic physician asked, "What have you done? Your cholesterol is so low which is the cause of a dangerous disorder!" Deeply concerned and frightened, I consulted a plant-based physician and asked many questions about my "*dangerous disorder.*" His response was, "Welcome to the plant-based world of great health!"

I was stupefied that a plant-based diet was the solution! It did not require prescriptions, supplements, or rigorous exercise. I was saving time and money, getting smarter, and losing weight. How could it be this easy to regain lost years of vibrant health and joy? I was devastated, and all I could do was weep. The answer had been under my nose all along! Food is powerful.

A **WFPB** *diet prevents inflammation* and reverses chronic disease. This information should be on TV stations, news channels, movie screens, and shouted from city street corners! Basic patient and human health education should be on billboards, the front pages of newspapers, *and* top stories on magazine covers at grocery stores. My enthusiasm was contagious and titanic. I could DO and BE anything with proper fuel.

Remember when smoking seemed normal? It took 25 years and 7,000 scientific studies before the U.S. government put a health-warning label on a box of cigarettes. When will the Surgeon General come to the rescue and warn you about the dangers of meat and cheese? Not in our lifetime! More people have died and will die from meat and dairy than all the deaths related to smoking! There's too much power and money in the beef and dairy industries, which influence poor legislative choices for the American people and our children. Wake up! Challenge your beliefs about food. Experience a beautiful transformation when you eat whole plants, organically grown by the sun, water and air!

There are 150-plus years of science-backed data and historical observations which support that plants reverse chronic disease. Chronic disease is crippling our country. Dr. Caldwell Esselstyn, from the Cleveland Clinic Heart Institute, promises that you will never have a second heart attack if you change your diet to a whole-food, plant-based diet. It took me 12 years of suffering, two trips to India, multiple diagnoses, and many prescriptions to accidentally discover the Truth.

Be a bullhorn for basic Health facts!

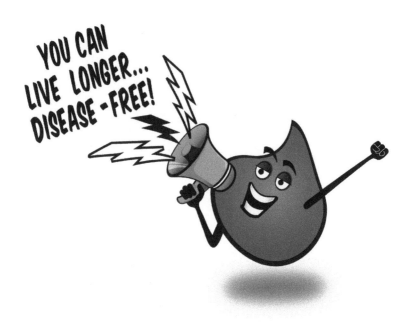

Healthy, energetic humans eat mostly plants, and science supports this. I took multiple, accredited courses in **WFPB** Nutrition including Cornell University's prestigious online class, "Plant-Based Nutrition" with Dr. Colin Campbell; the Plantrician's Project; the PCRM-International Nutrition Conference in Washington, D.C.; and several of Dr. John McDougall's online classes, including "The Starch Solution." I even went on a Wholistic Holiday Cruise and took 33 hours of lectures instead of swimming, tanning, and touring the Caribbean islands! In 2020, I completed the 18-day NEWSTART Program at Weimar, California.

After 230-plus hours of online and live classes and personally defeating metabolic syndrome, I created a class that followed my journey of discovering nature's food (plants), backed by research. My class, *"Truth in Food, The Blood Knows!"* challenged participants' to a 14-day plant-based diet. Before and after this challenge, participants' blood was tested. All participants had major improvements in their blood values; and they discovered how a plant-based diet heals both the body and the mind.

Your biggest challenge is ***believing*** and experiencing the truth, which is not financed by the beef and dairy industries, the FDA, and the Healthcare and Pharmaceutical Industries. There are no Broccoli Lobbyists fighting for your health in Washington, D.C. ***If you believe***, it is a matter of *life* and avoiding an early death. If you believe, the rest is history! The key to change is in your heart. Make a dramatic decision. It's time to stop suffering and begin true healing.

Change your Mind,

Change your Food,

Change your *Life*.

Mary Kay Matossian

3. Why are We so Confused?

More than anything, I want to astonish you with observational science, your personal experience, and facts that will change your life in an instant. This book is not all-encompassing with endless, tedious facts. We are too busy for that! I want to acknowledge and respect your time. When I experienced sudden and dramatic health improvements, a chain of reactions transformed my life.

'But first… What is your story? Why did you pick up this book? What do you want and need, and what do you deserve?

Take a moment, grab a pen and paper, and write your thoughts into your favorite journal. Think for a moment: Where do you get your information, and why do you believe that information? Who was the first person who told you, "Protein is everything!"? In your life, what authority continues with this narrative? Who gives you information, and why do you believe it? Here are stories from my life:

- I have bad genes; there is nothing I can do about that.

- Losing weight has been a lifelong losing battle.

- I have high blood pressure; it runs in my family.

- My mother had Alzheimer's at an early age; I'll have it too.

- I already know about great diets and food programs!

- What's a day without cheese? Are you kidding me?

- Every day is a good day for chicken-anything!

- I don't know who to believe; Everyone is so convincing!

- High protein, low protein, no carbs ... I give up!

- I have so much to lose; who do I believe?

- What is the actual cost of feeling lousy?

- What are the financial gains of feeling GREAT?

- I give more than I get; I feel resentful and tired.

- I'm irritable, anxious, and disappointed on a regular basis.

- Vitamins and prescriptions fix everything!

Whatever you have written in your journal, let's take a moment and acknowledge your beautiful story, including everything you know and everything you've been told. Our stories are heroic, gallant, sad, confusing, and frustrating. Let's rest our story for a moment. Confusion is our greatest enemy, the enemy that stops us in our tracks and prevents us from making great choices. Together, let's make room for another *story*, another set of rules, based on observational science and the truth that supports our sacred physiology.

There is no doubt that we live in a hostile food environment. All of us are suffering from a lack of knowledge! In this chapter, I discuss the gloomy statistics about our health and the glitches in the health care system that keeps us misinformed. How sick are we, and why?

After years of suffering from metabolic syndrome, I realized it was due to a high animal protein diet. You couldn't convince me to eat less protein. I was "doing my job and I was doing my body good!" Bacon and eggs for breakfast, raw salmon sushi for lunch, and grilled chicken for dinner. But I felt lousy, and I needed real answers. What I discovered is that a low-protein, plant-based diet *extends* life! Chapter 6 thoroughly explores the science behind eliminating animal-based proteins and animal-based fats from your meals.

Genetics are also important, but genetics only represent a potential for disease. Our food choices open or close genetic opportunity! Our genes come with us at birth, and we cannot control that. What we can control is what we put in our mouths. Smoking, alcohol, and the Standard American Diet rich in beef and dairy, loaded with "bad-gene" hormones awaken cancers and diseases. So you have the power to say good-bye to bad genes.

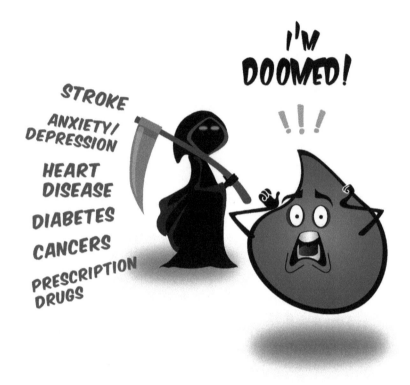

Chapter 7 explores the world of complex carbohydrates. We discover the simple solution to metabolic syndrome: Reduce inflammation.

The better we understand ourselves, the better we manage life's extremes. Do you wonder when things are going to get "back to normal"? Do you wonder when things are going to slow down? Extremes are the new normal. Our lives are more stressful than ever! *The Economist* and *Forbes Magazine* said:

"2019 is the Year of the Vegan."

More than at any other time, we must be skilled and empowered to navigate our lives and help those around us. Start by choosing your food wisely. Simple foods like the baked potato, steamed vegetables, and a fresh green salad fill us with nutrients, provide extended energy, and calm our minds because they do not contain bacterial toxins. Chapter 7 explores how food impacts our emotions and intelligence. Are you ready to reverse metabolic syndrome for good? Let's start!

In 2014, I was desperate to know everything there was to know about great health: How to lose weight; how to live a long, happy and productive life; and how to be patient, resilient and conquer daily stress. For years, I spent hundreds of dollars on magazines at grocery stores and newsstands, reading about the latest and greatest recommendation on what foods and vitamins give us the biggest bang for our buck. Every year, I read the Mayo Clinic's New Year's Journal on the "latest research" on health, cancer, diabetes, Alzheimer's, and heart disease. Yes, I was well-informed. However, the data from all these different authorities on health and wellness did not add up. Recently, a study revealed that most physicians get their nutritional information from the same glossy magazines that we do! Sadly, everyone is baffled, including healthcare professionals.

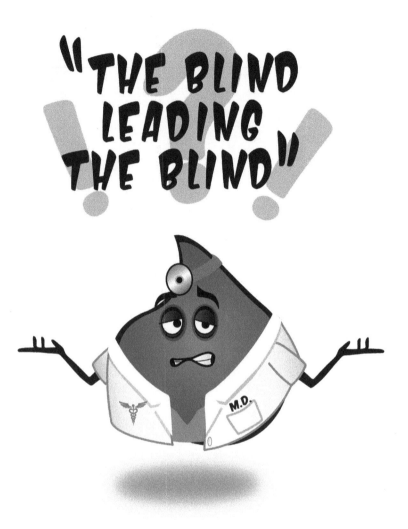

Let me ask you a question: What do *you* do when you are confused? Who among us **_LOVES_** being confused when it comes to major decisions in our lives? Here are examples of everyday decisions: Are you ever confused about which side of the highway you should drive on? Are you ever confused about touching a rattlesnake or hugging a grizzly bear in the wild? Are you ever confused about drinking cyanide or arsenic to see how they taste? Humans intuitively do not like to get injured, poisoned, or killed. When it comes to survival, know the basic *rules* to survive and thrive!

Many years ago, my four-year-old son would come running into the house crying because a bumblebee had stung him. This happened repeatedly! Finally, I asked him, "What are you doing to get stung by a bumblebee over and over again?"

His response was remarkable: "Mom, they're so fuzzy and cute; I'm just holding him!"

When we know the rules of how to survive and not get hurt, we are motivated to follow those rules.

Then, why are we so confused about our health and what to eat? The beef and dairy industries pull in $100,000,000,000 in profits per year; that's one-hundred billion dollars. Each year, they spend $101,000,000 on marketing ads to promote animal products; that is one-hundred million dollars annually to confuse our food choices for corporate gain. This diet, high in animal cholesterol, is handed to us from before birth, in utero, from our mothers. This diet that "does a body good" has been around for 150 years. Clearly, this diet harms us, but our subconscious minds kick in, and we eat it anyway.

Talking about food these days is like talking about abortion rights. With all the conflicting information, political tension, global warming, and millions of dollars spent on marketing what to eat that we're bombarded with these days, no wonder we are confused! When we are confused.... We do nothing and continue doing the same thing, even if it's harmful. We have information overload, and the message of food is deep in our subconscious. Brain fog, stress, chronic pain, and fatigue prevent us from making good choices. We continue to eat harmful foods because we are tired. You deserve better: a better brain, a better body, and better health. You deserve the truth. We are hardwired to win, survive, thrive and avoid an early death.

How Sick Are We?

We are the richest democracy in the world, but at the same time we are the sickest people in the world. Yes, I was one of those sick people. Our healthcare system is extremely expensive. We all know someone who does not have healthcare insurance; who does not qualify for Medicaid because they make "too much money." We cringe at what they are going through and wonder how they are financing their medical bills. Have you noticed Americans are sicker ... sooner? Each of us knows someone who has heart disease, early-onset Alzheimer's, diabetes, cancer, depression, and autoimmune disorders. By the time we go to the doctor, we already have significant damage to our blood circulation, and major chronic disease is already onboard with troubling symptoms.

The U.S. healthcare system is designed to treat symptoms, *not* prevent disease. Our system should be called "Sickness Care." The U.S. healthcare system has its *head* in the sand, and the system is making a lot of money from our suffering and financial losses! The current annual healthcare cost is 20 percent of the U.S. GDP. We spend $3.5 trillion on healthcare use per year! Its focus is on expensive prescription drugs, surgery, medical procedures, and chemotherapy. Here are a few concerning statistics:

- One out of every four deaths in the U.S. is due to cancer (American Cancer Association)

- One of three Americans have type 2 diabetes (American Diabetes Association)

- 70 percent of all Americans are overweight; Thin is Abnormal!

- The sixth cause of death is taking prescriptions *correctly*. That's 100,000 deaths!

- Seventeen million people worldwide die each year from heart attacks. (American Heart Association) ***That's double New York City's population!***

These are frightening statistics; and the underlying cause of these statistics is ***chronic inflammation***, damages our blood circulation system. Life expectancy in the United States has been declining since 2014. The last population decline was in 1918, after the great Spanish flu pandemic.

For example, if you have diabetes, you are probably overweight and you have high blood pressure! For these conditions, you are taking several medications which have dangerous side effects. If you are waiting for blood test results due to a cancer scare, you may be getting ready for your first heart attack. This sounds sarcastic, but with deep sadness, this is the American Plight. These statistics are widespread and terrifying! You can catch an early death in the United States the way you can catch the common cold or COVID-19! Who needs this?

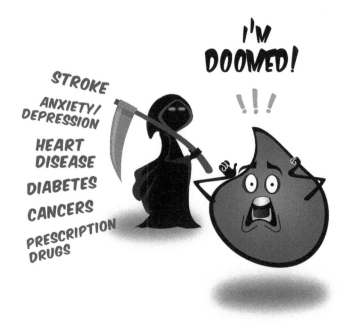

The worst part is that enormous nonprofit organizations including the American Cancer Association, the American Diabetes Association, and the American Heart Association are largely silent about the cause of these common deaths. American corporations are likewise culprits in the healthcare crisis of silence. Keeping us sick, uninformed, and fed with toxic, cheap food keeps profits high in all industries. Stop this pandemic of early death and reverse chronic conditions today!

Dr. Michael Greger, who authored the book, *How Not to Die*, claims that most diseases which cause death are related to *food*. In fact, 70 percent of all deaths are related to chronic diseases of our own making. What will your life look like if you change your food now? You deserve better, and I have great news for you! Hang in there with me.

I'M YOUR BLOOD
&
I NEED YOU!

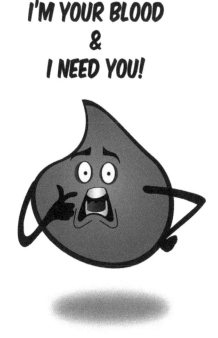

ACLS – A Healthcare Solution… Really?

One of the reasons I went to nursing school was to serve. In the early 1980s, nurses had only a few patients. We doted over our patients and holistically cared for them for our entire shifts. By the end of my shift, my patients came alive with hope, joy, and determination to get better! As part of my career, education goals, and to serve my patients better, I took the ACLS Class. ACLS is the Advanced Cardiac Life Support class, which is required for emergency room physicians, surgeons, cardiologists, operating room nurses, and ICU nurses. This class teaches healthcare providers how to stop a heart attack while it's happening, outside *or* in a hospital. It requires a knowledge of multiple drugs, operating the AED heart-start machine, and the rigorous pumping of the chest to re-start the heart manually. For 10 years, I successfully took this class for re-certification. I was ready anytime, anywhere, to save a Life! My goal was to be of service, in a hospital or out of a hospital, to anyone, anywhere…

However, the last time I took the ACLS class, I noticed a disclosure in small print. Most heart attacks are *not stopped or prevented* with ACLS Training. In fact, 90 percent of *all* cardiac arrest victims *die* outside of a hospital despite the presence of highly trained personnel. Cardiac arrest means the heart has stopped beating and blood circulation stops as well. Without immediate correction and restarting the heart, the victim will die. If you have a heart attack *in* a hospital, there's a 75 percent chance of death despite the use of the ACLS technique with I.V. medications, the AED heart-start machine, and a team of highly trained physicians and nurses. When I discovered this statistic, I was shocked that my ACLS skills were almost meaningless! Who would take a Life & Death skills class that guarantees a 90-percent failure rate? A 90-percent failure rate means your patient will die 90 percent of the time.

Thus, if you have heart disease and you are at risk of having a heart attack, ACLS will not save you. It is time for a *food* change that guarantees a 100-percent success rate. World-wide, 17 million people die annually from heart attacks; that's double New York City's population! This is major *news*! Heart attacks occur in countries where dairy and animal products are a major part of the diet. You will *NOT* have a heart attack if you do not eat meat and cheese. Heart attacks are nearly 100 percent preventable if you avoid animal products.

During World War II, German troops occupied Norway and they took the Norwegians' livestock for themselves. During this time, the Norwegians were left with nothing but potatoes and turnips! This was an extremely stressful time for the Norwegians; however, heart disease in Norway plummeted. Shortly after the war, the Norwegians regained access to their livestock and continued with their high beef and dairy consumption. Heart disease after World War II skyrocketed again. History and science support the rapid impact food has on heart disease.

How Many Medications Are You Taking?

Patients with metabolic syndrome will have heartburn, indigestion, and constipation. These are common conditions. Omeprazole and ranitidine are prescribed for indigestion and reflux disorders. Laxatives are prescribed regularly to help alleviate the lack of fiber in your diet and to compensate for all the side effects from the other medications you are taking. Sound familiar? You are now on more than 10 medications. You are advised to "eat healthy" and lose weight, and are scheduled for a return doctor visit in one or two months ... *great!* The American healthcare system is the best in the world at diagnosis and treatment, but it does not address the root cause of most medical conditions.

When it comes to prevention and healing, there's enormous room for improvement. U.S. corporate healthcare systems allow for just enough time for a quick, 15-minute diagnosis and a few prescriptions to treat the problem. You deserve better.

Healthcare providers are not
Educated on the LINK between
FOOD and Chronic disease.

This lack of knowledge benefits the pharmaceutical industry, which has a pill for every condition and a pill for every side effect to **other pills**! When a patient visits a physician, "It's the blind leading the blind in healing"! If healthcare providers are not practicing healthy behaviors, how can they teach healthy behaviors to their patients? It's time for a new plan. Diseases and prescriptions are ravaging our bodies and our minds, inflicting enormous suffering. Most diagnoses are of illnesses that are preventable and reversible on diet alone. You deserve better.

The Standard American Diet (**_SAD_**) is the biggest healthcare crisis because people are needlessly suffering and dying prematurely from preventable and reversible diseases. Food gets us into trouble, and food has the power to get us out of trouble and change the direction of our nation's health and the health of the world, and reverse climate damage. A **_WFPB_** diet has the power to reverse existing disease and begin true healing. The human body has an incredible ability to heal itself if only it is given the opportunity to do so. Instead of poisoning ourselves with each and every meal, every three to four hours with meat and cheese, a plant-based diet allows for a dramatic transformation to reverse disease and heal our bodies and our minds.

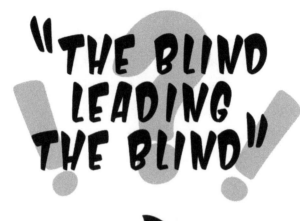

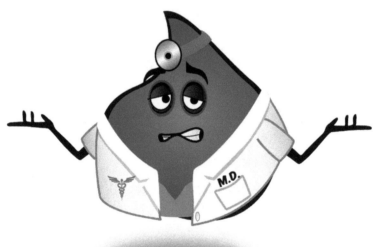

4. You Need Your Superpowers!

Who has your back? Your family members, parents, friends, your spouse, the village, and/or the U.S. government? Are you sure? Who really has your back? ***It is your responsibility to have your back.*** You may be in a place where you are the only one pursuing a diet change. You are alone and you may feel unsupported… Do it anyway! Less than 2 percent of the U.S. population chooses to eat whole plants. The Food Movement is a slow, arduous movement, and it is not going away! The most difficult and inconvenient things you have to do in your life, you do alone. We are natural pioneers for a better life. We will do whatever it takes to help loved ones and future generations.

When I changed my food from the Standard American Diet to whole plants, something changed inside of me. I fell in *love* with how food made me feel. The connection is clear: What we eat matters. My heart and my awareness expanded. My crusty paradigm of rigid beliefs dissolved. A larger, more compassionate life emerged. When I look around, there is a sea of needless suffering. When a stranger is unkind to me, I automatically think, "It must be what they had for lunch; or did they skip breakfast?" My compassion continues to grow and expand. Sometimes, I need to rest in sadness and grief. Living the whole food, plant-based lifestyle is a matter of life and death. My health improved so quickly. Abundance, calmness, intelligence, and my gratitude soared. Through meet-ups, I met innovative and forward-thinking people. Public opinion is changing. Intuitively, you move away from meat and cheese as your vitality soars. Are you ready to be a part of the people's movement that could help every American and every hungry person on the planet? Join us and be a part of the solution.

Our typical American patient, suffering from metabolic syndrome and fatty liver disease, enters the health care system begging for help. The doctor will *not* discuss the impacts of food on their health. This is the ONLY reason I authored this book. Give the whole food plant-based diet a try! Form a vegan support group; get together monthly and share meals, recipes, and successes. Encourage each other on this journey of healing and self-discovery with a transformed body and mind.

What happens if our typical patient follows the doctor's advice, takes all medications properly, without changing his or her diet? The patient, on an animal-based diet, will spiral downhill with progressively deteriorating and complicated health problems. A tragic health event such as a stroke, heart attack, cancer, Alzheimer's, renal failure, and cirrhosis will shorten the patient's lifespan. However, these health problems are preventable and reversible.

On the contrary, those who switch to a plant-based diet begin the healing process within days. The plant-based diet gives the typical American patient with metabolic syndrome the *power* to break the chains of suffering and prevent early death. Do yourself a favor. Choose foods that promote healing and survival! The power is in your hands!

Did you know it takes 1,000 gallons of water to produce one pound of ground beef? Yet there are water restrictions all over California and across the globe! You cannot water your lawn in California, but you can buy as much ground beef as you want there. How many gallons of water does the beef and dairy industries use across the globe, including toxic runoff? California is on fire annually, and it's scary. When I changed my diet, my life changed.

October 8, 2017, was the best day of my life! I conquered my fear of public speaking and taught my very first class, "Truth in Food, the Blood Knows!" I took several photos of my home that day because it looked like my home was robbed and ransacked! My kitchen, dining room and living room had pots, pans, coffee machines, folders, papers, books, and leftover food everywhere. I went to bed that night happy, joyful, as I embarked on my mission to educate anyone who would listen!

At 2:10 a.m., Monday morning, October 9, 2017, I abruptly woke up because I was perspiring. My husband was out of town, and I was alone. The house was shaking, and the winds were howling! I was extremely hot and sweaty on that chilly October morning. My house was incredibly warm. Suddenly, I was awake, and I pulled out my earplugs and looked around. There was an unfamiliar bright orange glow and I wondered, "Are these new emergency lights?" It was quiet except the howling winds. A bitter-sweet caramel odor filled the air, "Aha! It's an electrical fire somewhere in the house," I thought. No big deal; I would put it out. When I entered my adjoining bathroom, the upper windows hosted an inferno. The trees outside were on fire and slamming against the upper windows! This could not be happening…"Wake up!" I ran toward my bedroom balcony and pushed the curtains away. To my shock, there were 10-foot-high flames surrounding my deck, with no way for me to escape. It was silent. "Where are the sirens, the police, the firetrucks? Has my imagination gone wild?" I thought.

Dread overcame me as I ran into my living room. My beautiful home was surrounded by fire and I was stuck inside. Fire was dancing in every window: The kitchen, the dining room, and the living room, and the front door was hot! Desperate, I ran into the garage to open the garage doors … no response. The electricity was off, and the garage doors were hot. The wind was slamming the fire against the garage doors. If I opened the garage doors, I knew the inferno would rush in and blind me and set our two cars ablaze. I felt like I was in "The Hunger Games," navigating an escape that was clearly a matter of life or death. If this was real, I had no choice but to escape on foot.

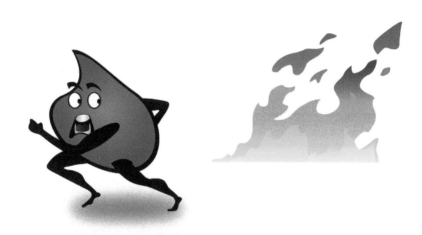

WHEN YOU CHANGE YOUR FOOD-
YOU CHANGE YOUR JOURNEY

What Do You Need to Survive a Raging Fire?

I will never forget those moments of being alone inside my burning house, left behind and forgotten. No one was coming to my rescue. I stood inside my burning home, surrounded by fire. I had a choice: Panic or think. The hillside across the street was ablaze and flames were coming down the hillside rapidly. My garage doors were on fire and I could not access either of our cars. Every tree surrounding my suburban home was on fire, and the 60-mile-per-hour winds were blowing the fire in every direction. "This is a firestorm!" As I stood in the middle of my living room surrounded by fire, it was the longest *pause* of my life.

Believing in what I was seeing and experiencing was a matter of life or death. No one was coming to my rescue. My entire neighborhood was engulfed in fire, and I was left behind. There were no sirens.

Because of my formal education in nursing, it was clear to me that burning alive was a terrible way to die. I had to *escape and believe* in my survival. I made the decision to get out. What would shield me from the sheets of fire going in every direction?

We operated a Surgery Center in Northern California and we were part of the 11-county disaster plan, from Oakland to Humboldt Counties. We met with firefighters annually and we reviewed what went wrong with the Oakland Fires of 1999. Like an encyclopedia, my brain fed me the tools to survive. Without changing my pajamas, I shoved on running shoes without socks and grabbed a raincoat. A raincoat protects against droplets of rain, and I knew it would protect me from sheets of fire going upward. My hair could catch on fire, so I pulled on the hood of my raincoat. It was a firestorm, and the winds were directing the fire everywhere! The only thing I grabbed was my cell phone and a thread of hope. There was no obvious way out. Everything was left behind, except my cell phone.

I ran down the back deck and got ready to jump over the railing. Abruptly I stopped when I saw eight-foot-high flames beneath the deck. Those flames were taller than me! Jumping into a fire did not seem like a promising idea. As I backed away from the corner of the upper deck, I focused on getting to the Fountaingrove Golf Course. The golf course was the only thing not burning, but a brush fire was blocking my way. "This is my only chance!" With my eyes closed and my hooded raincoat covering my hair, I ran as fast as I could and slammed into a big rock. I fell facedown into the grass, which was cool to the touch and still green. Scrambling back to my feet, I ran like the wind across the golf course and looked over my shoulder. All my neighbors' homes were burning down. As I crossed the golf course, a creek, and into solid six-foot fence, I could hardly breathe. The oxygen was sucked out of the air by the flames, and the smoke was as thick as a wool blanket. Fortunately, the fence I ran into collapsed, and I stumbled into the middle of the street. Through the dark, gray haze of toxic smoke appeared a police trooper and the last fire truck searching for fire victims. I was one of the last people out of the Fountaingrove neighborhood alive. The fires burned for weeks. Forty people died and 10,000 structures were destroyed in Sonoma and Napa Counties. At the time, it was the worst fire in California history, but now every year is the worst fire year in California history. The story goes on.

My body and mind were there for me. That week, more than 40 people died, many from my neighborhood. It is a heartbreaking tragedy I will never forget. Just a year earlier, I had been overweight, taking sleeping pills, and suffering from brain fog, depression, and metabolic syndrome. My mind was clear of excess cholesterol. Like an encyclopedia, my mind guided me through this hellacious event. We lost everything in that home, but I was spared a violent and agonizing death. I am grateful to the plant-based diet that saved my life in more ways than one.

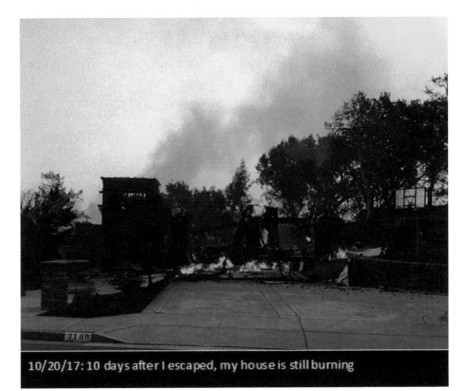

10/20/17: 10 days after I escaped, my house is still burning

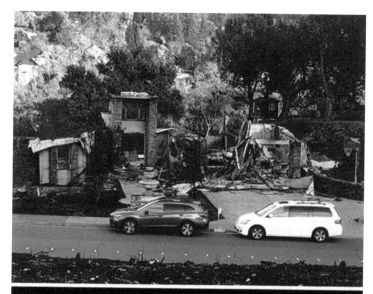

Three weeks after fire of 10/9/2017.

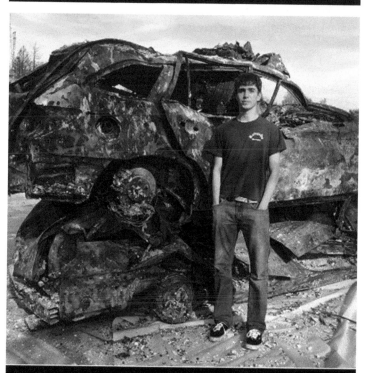

Thanksgiving 2017: Subaru Outback and Honda Pilot.

During my escape from the Santa Rosa Fires of 2017, I inhaled massive amounts of toxic smoke. When I was at the police department, I exhaled deeply, and black smoke came out of my lungs. The hospitals were shut down and off-limits to healthy-sick people like me, so I chose to get weekly acupuncture to clear my lungs. A week later, as I sat on the acupuncture table, I began to weep.

The acupuncturist asked, "Are you crying because you feel abandoned and forgotten?"

My response was, "No, I've never felt so loved, cared for, and lucky to be alive."

Her response was, "Ah, your heart is breaking because it is getting bigger with gratitude!"

Yes. The community came together, helped its fire victims, and it continues to rebuild.

The WFPB gave me the clarity of mind, strength in body, and the *belief* to survive and thrive during and after the fire. This is my story. ***No one came to my rescue during the fire***. After much speculation and two years, my husband and I moved for the seventh and final time to Reno, Nevada. Being prepared for a crisis in body and in mind changed my life. Consuming healthy, whole, plant-based foods, feeling grateful and believing in my ability to survive was a matter of life or death.

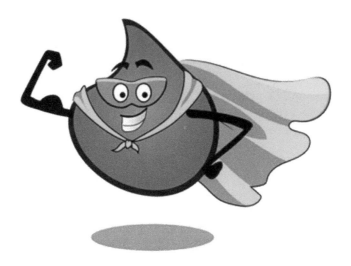

Mary Kay Matossian

5. Reboot Your Blood!

B y now, it should be understood that what we eat has everything to do with our health and the health of our blood. Blood is our great warrior and protects us daily, never stopping until our last breath. Almost 2,500 years ago, Hippocrates said:

"Let food be thy Medicine and Let Medicine be thy food!"

Hippocrates knew something that we have forgotten today. For several years, I was a biometrics wellness nurse, and went into different corporations in Northern California. A team of nurses would meet with healthy employees and check their biometrics: Blood pressure, BMI, and basic blood values such as total cholesterol, triglycerides, lipids, and blood glucose. If participants' blood glucose was high, we tested their hemoglobin **A1C**. Blood values for many "healthy employees" were abnormal. Our job was to give basic information on "eat right, eat less, and exercise." Our advice was obscure. Many employees were embarrassed by their abnormal bloodwork numbers, and they knew they could "do better" but didn't know how. To this day, it saddens me that I had misinformation, and we didn't have the correct answers to help corporate employees improve their bloodwork numbers.

After I became meat- and cheese-free, I filled up on beans, potatoes, and steamed vegetables! I noticed a marked improvement in my blood results, and I felt fantastic! As I continued with my job as a biometrics wellness nurse, I gave participants gentle but firm advice on avoiding meat and cheese. Plants do not contain unwanted harmful cholesterol. The nutrients and antioxidants in plants fight for our wellbeing. Just like other animals, we make our own cholesterol. On rare occasions, a participant would have blood results that were astonishing! I would ask, "Are you vegan?" *Yes,* was always the answer! These vegans had normal cholesterol levels of 130 mg/dl. Their blood pressure would be 100/60. Their fasting blood glucose was below 95, and their BMI was often below 24.

What Is Total Cholesterol?

First of all, blood values are confidential! Do not share your bloodwork with anyone unless you fully trust that person. You do not need to explain, share or justify your bloodwork to coworkers, friends, or anyone. Quite often, routine bloodwork reveals underlying disease, and catches participants by surprise! We always respect every participant's privacy, and recommend additional bloodwork by their primary care physicians.

Total **_cholesterol_** measures fatty substances in your blood. Too much cholesterol sticks to the walls of your arteries, causing plaque to build up, narrowing your arteries. This causes blood pressure to rise, which can lead to stroke and heart disease. Too much cholesterol comes from meat, fish, cheese, chicken, milk, and eggs. The ideal total cholesterol value should be less than 200 mg/dl.

What Are Triglycerides?

Triglycerides are the most common fat floating in the blood. When we eat highly processed foods and fatty animal products, they are immediately converted to triglycerides by the liver. Excess calories, converted to triglycerides, are stored along the inner lining of arteries, which leads to the formation of plaque. Triglyceride values should be less than 150 mg/dl. The human body was not meant to consume a diet rich in animal products.

What Are High- and Low-Density Lipids?

These lipids are complete opposites! High-density lipids are "**_Happy Fats_**" that digest and clear away low-density lipids or "**_Lousy Fats_**." High-density lipids digest and eliminate low-density lipids through the liver. Low-density lipids (Lousy Fats) are waxy and sticky, just like cheesecake! Low-density lipids become **PLAQUE** inside arteries, causing coronary artery disease. Plaque blocks blood flow, oxygen, and nutrients from getting to the heart and brain. Plaque prevents micro-circulation, and it comes from meat, cheese and dairy. Plaque-formation is not a result of bad genes, but of poor food choices. Ideal values for low-density lipids are those less than 130 mg/dl.

Societies in other parts of the world, such as rural Africa and rural China, do not have heart disease, osteoporosis, or breast cancer because they eat a plant-based diet, free of animal products. However, if these people relocate to the United States and adopt the Standard American Diet (**SAD**), they become sick immediately with chronic diseases. Now is the time for change.

High density lipids (Happy Fats) protect against stroke, diabetes-2, heart disease, high blood pressure, and high cholesterol. Exercise, walking, and deep breathing increase this lipid! Yikes! Hard work and your homework. We want high-density lipids to be above 60 mg/dl, which is rare! When we change our diet to a low-fat, whole-food, plant-based diet and combine this diet with daily walks, high-density lipids increase.

What Is Blood Glucose?

Glucose is the simple carbohydrate that the body uses for energy to the brain and muscle cells. Complex carbohydrates break down to the one and only simple carbohydrate, GLUCOSE. With the help of insulin, glucose leaves the blood and enters into brain and muscle cells. However, when total cholesterol and triglycerides are too high, these large fat cells trap insulin! Glucose can't get out of the blood and glucose begins to rise in the blood. This is the cause of Diabetes-2. Glucose can't get to the muscles or brain cells.

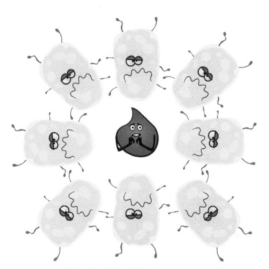

OUR BODY HAS AN UNLIMITED CAPACITY TO STORE FAT IN THE ABDOMEN & LIVER CAUSING FATTY LIVER DISEASE.

For example, suppose you are thirsty, and you need a glass of water, but you have duct tape across your mouth. There is no getting water into your body with your mouth taped! This is how diabetes-2 works! Water is like glucose. Water can't get into the body because duct tape is blocking the mouth. Glucose can't get to the muscle cells because cholesterol is blocking the insulin from getting glucose into the muscles. Diabetes-2 is *not* a disease of too much *sugar*, but a disease of too much *fat* which causes Insulin-resistance. Fasting blood glucose should be less than 95 mg/dl, and if you're not fasting less than 140 mg/dl. If your blood glucose is over 200 mg/dl, you have diabetes.

I'M YOUR BLOOD
&
I NEED YOU!

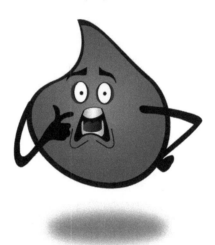

What Is Hemoglobin, A1C?

With a drop of blood, A1CNow is a simple test that measures the average blood glucose levels over a 90-day period. Hemoglobin is the protein in red blood cells, and hemoglobin carries oxygen in the blood. Glucose attaches to hemoglobin, and it becomes glycated. If there is too much glucose in the bloodstream, hemoglobin becomes extra glycated! The lifespan of a red blood cell is approximately 90 days. Through this process of glycation, the hemoglobin reveals the average blood glucose levels over the course of

90 days. Normal A1C is between 4–6. A1C levels above 7 indicate diabetes.

Stop! There is a phenomenon that occurs when you stop eating animal products. Your blood cholesterol level may initially go up because the toxic fat re-enters the bloodstream from fat storage and plaques along the arteries. Cholesterol leaves the body through the liver and lungs! Ultimately, your lipids will go down in a short period of time. Did you know that when you lose 10 pounds of fat, eight pounds leave the body through breathing. The other two pounds leave the body through urine, sweat, and fecal waste!

What's High Blood Pressure?

A diet high in salt, prepared foods, alcohol, meat, dairy, and seafood, combined with stress, contributes to high blood pressure. We need around 400 mg of sodium per day, which we get from vegetables and grains! However, we typically take in 4,000 mg of sodium per day! Massive sodium intake is poisonous, and stiffens our blood vessels, pulling in excess fluid from outside the bloodstream. We become thirsty and dehydrated. Excess salt-intake causes high blood pressure and chronic dehydration. Blood pressure is the silent killer. Get salt out of your diet. Sumac, a dark purple berry that tastes like *salt*, is a great salt substitute. Sumac makes giving up salt easier! *Sumac* can be ordered on Amazon.

Your bloodwork is a snapshot of how you're doing at that moment. When you change your food, your bloodwork improves rapidly!

Rename Your Food

The power is within you to make these changes. Plant foods are delicious and filling, and they are available everywhere, including your own kitchen! Here's an interesting story: You meet a new and interesting lady in town, and she is very excited to get to know *you* better. She invites you over to her new house and prepares for you her favorite smoothie. She states that it tastes delicious, and feels good when it hits your stomach. It won national awards, and she is famous for her smoothies! She insists you must drink the whole smoothie in order to get the benefits of it. She also confesses that she never hears from her new friends again after sharing her amazing smoothie with them. She doesn't make the connection and insists that this smoothie will change your life! ingredient is **CYANIDE**…. Eek!

So what do you do? Do you drink the whole smoothie in order to save a new and exciting friendship? Do you risk embarrassing yourself or her? She is insistent that you must drink the whole thing! What do you do? When I initially ask this question in my classes, many participants get a suspicious look in their eyes. Everyone knows ingesting **CYANIDE** will cause an agonizing, abrupt death! What is the matter with this new friend? You want to foster that new friendship, but not drink the poison. Your decision is thus crystal clear: No matter how curious you become, you will *never* "taste" *cyanide* or *arsenic*! Correct? It's like kissing a rattlesnake or hugging a grizzly bear. Humans do not like to get hurt or catastrophically injured.

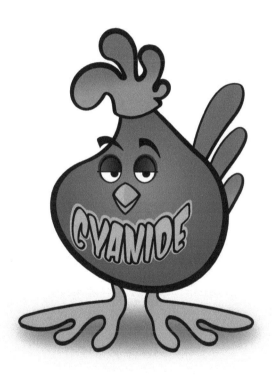

The challenge of becoming whole-food, plant-based in terms diet got a whole lot easier when I renamed my food. Meat and cheese will always harm you. Re-name the foods that harm you! No matter the temptation, we'd never taste *cyanide* just because it looks, tastes, and smells good.

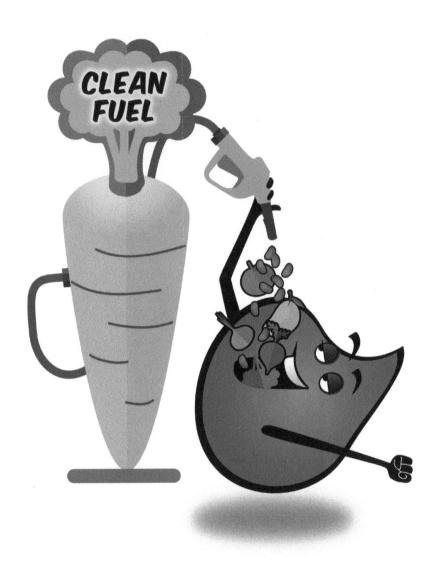

Total Cholesterol: A measure of fatty substances in your blood. Too much cholesterol builds plaque in your arteries and blocks blood flow, which increases the risk of stroke and heart disease. Too much cholesterol comes from meat, fish, cheese, chicken, milk and eggs.

- Ideal: -200 mg/dl
- At Risk: +200 mg/dl

Triglycerides: Excess food and calories are converted to triglycerides by the liver, and they are the most common fat floating in the blood. Then, it's stored in fat cells everywhere in the body!

- Ideal: -200 mg/dl
- At Risk: +200 mg/dl

High Density Lipids: "Happy" cholesterol removes "Lousy" cholesterol from artery and blood vessel walls, and protects against stroke and heart disease. Walking Increases this lipid!

- Ideal: -200 mg/dl
- At Risk: +200 mg/dl

Low Density Lipids: "Lousy" cholesterol is bad! It's like warm cheesecake; it is thick and waxy, and causes coronary artery disease. It comes from the FOOD we EAT! NOT our genes.

- Ideal: -200 mg/dl
- At Risk: +200 mg/dl

Blood Glucose: Provides energy to the brain and the muscles! High cholesterol (traveling fat) BLOCKS Insulin from getting glucose to the brain and muscles. Glucose is trapped in the blood! Cholesterol wraps around insulin and PREVENTS it from getting glucose to the brain and muscles!

- Ideal: -200 mg/dl
- At Risk: +200 mg/dl

HIGH Fiber grabs Cholesterol and walks it out
Of the body!!

6. Protein IS the Problem!

T he greatest health study in the history of mankind is the China Study. Chou En-Lai, the Premier of China in 1949–1976, was furious because he was dying of cancer, and he did not know why. In the 1970s, he ordered a survey of his 880,000,000 citizens, collecting data on who died of what and where they lived in China. Between 1988and 2008, Cornell University, with Dr. Collin Campbell, Oxford University, and the Chinese Academy of Medicine, discovered more than 2,300 points of data, patterns, and correlations that revealed a shocking and undeniable connection between *food* and *death*:

> ***"The higher your animal protein intake,***
> ***the greater your cancer risk and***
> ***the shorter your lifespan….!"***

Chou En-Lai died before he discovered why he had cancer. He ate seafood every day. The regions whose populations consumed a diet high in fish and animal products had a 10,000-percent increased risk of *cancer* compared to the rural, inland areas whose populations did not have access to seafood and animal products. It was a

100-fold difference! If a Chinese person moved to a different region, they gradually acquired the cancer risks of that region because their food choices *changed*. The Chinese who ate the least amount of animal protein, less than 40 grams per day, lived the longest lives.

The magnitude of the China Study is critically acclaimed because China was geographically and genetically stable up until 2008. For example, where you were born is where you lived, worked, raised your family, and died. There was minimal mobility during this time. Therefore, China had few scientific variables. No one was entering China, and no one was leaving. China's gene pool was homogenous throughout the country for thousands of years. The China Study is the *purest*, most accurate observational study on earth, surveying 880 million people! The correlation between food and chronic disease *is* undeniable. The time is *now*. Believing in a plant-based diet is a matter of life and death.

What Is Protein?

Protein is a chain of amino acids, which are building blocks for muscles and cell repair. Stomach acid breaks down proteins to single amino acids. There are 20 amino acids; of these, eight are "essential," meaning we get these amino acids by simply eating food. Amino acids are stored in the liver and readily available like books in a library! When we need certain amino acids, our bodies pull them from the liver-library. Your liver generates thousands of proteins for your body's needs daily. According to the China

Study, and several other studies, humans need 20 to 30 grams of protein per day. Your liver *recycles* amino acids and creates thousands of proteins exclusively for your body! Your liver loves you!

Vegetables are surprisingly high in protein, nutrients, minerals, and fiber without the harmful effects of animal-based cholesterol. One-hundred percent of your protein needs can come from plants. Per pound, plants contain more protein than animal products! Spinach, kale, and broccoli are 40 percent protein by weight, while chicken and beef are only 26 percent protein by weight (see the picture below for more information). Animal proteins shorten your lifespan, but proteins from plants lengthen your lifespan and protect against cancers and all chronic disease. Deadly animal-based toxins are cholesterol, bacterial protein toxins, Trimethylamine N-oxide (TMAO), and the hormone Insulin Growth Factor-1 (IGF-1), which promotes all forms of cancer.

By the way, "protein deficiency" ONLY exists in conditions of starvation such as anorexia nervosa or living in a region of the world suffering from famine. If you're consuming under 400 calories per day, you will have protein deficiency.

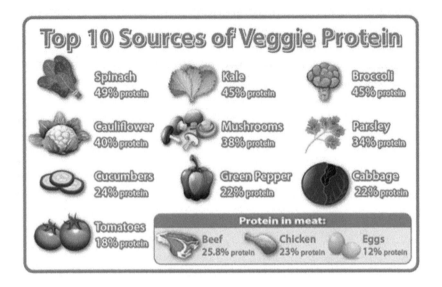

Animal Protein Harms Our Bodies

Consuming animal proteins, such as cheese and meat, create an acidic and inflammatory response. Remember, adult bodies only need 20 to 30 grams of protein per day. Those who follow the Atkins, or ketogenic, diet take in 200 grams of animal protein per day. *That's tenfold!* Animal proteins make our blood acidic, which increases inflammation and promotes chronic disease. Blood is alkaline, with a pH of between 7.35 and 7.45. If our blood becomes too acidic, however, *we die.* Your blood travels to every cell in your body, getting rid of toxins, and supplying nutrients to vital organs. Our blood is our greatest ally, regulator, and warrior. However, after a lifetime of consuming animal products and toxins, the blood is defeated and struggles with supporting pH balance and fighting constant inflammation. How does the body get rid of toxins?

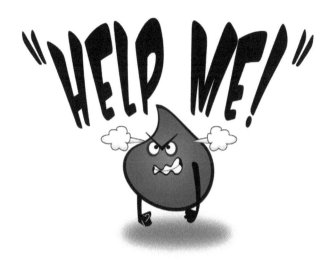

How Did My Bones Get into My Kidneys?

Animal products make our blood acidic! Our stomach produces extra hydrochloric acid to break down animal proteins, which cause excess acid production. Remember, blood is alkaline and it is our greatest warrior!

Do you remember the "flushing kits" from science classrooms in high school science labs? When a student accidentally got a mild acid on their skin, they had to flush their skin with water and rinse the acid off. Typically, a burn or red spot is left behind, and the skin heals. Our blood has the same mechanism. After a high-protein, acidic meal, extra fluid flushes the acid out of our blood system. The extra fluid leaves our body through the kidneys. After a salty, fatty, high-protein meal, we feel thirsty! The blood is constantly grabbing extra fluid from our body, and this makes our skin become dry and wrinkled at a young age.

When our blood is acidic, it steals calcium bicarbonate from our bones to neutralize excess acid resulting from eating beef and dairy. This "flushing process" is called homeostasis. Once the blood is neutralized, the calcium bicarbonate, from our bones, has nowhere to go and it cannot go back to the bones. Instead, the calcium bicarbonate leaves the body through the kidneys and urination. Calcium bicarbonate gets *stuck* in the kidney filters, accumulates, and begins to form kidney stones!

Calcium is critical for bodily function, so where do we get calcium? Calcium is a mineral found in soil. As plants grow, they pull calcium into their stems, and calcium is incorporated into the plant. Just as a cow eats grass, by eating a plant-based diet we absorb all the calcium and essential minerals needed for healthy bones. We do not need a middleman, the cow, to meet our calcium needs. In fact, the strongest animals on the planet are herbivores, eating only plants. These herbivores are the bull elephant, the gorilla, the thoroughbred horse, the hippopotamus, the giraffe, etc.

A diet high in animal protein creates inflammation and dehydration! Calcium is constantly leaving our bones to neutralize the blood, and it exits our bodies through the kidneys. Our bones get lighter and lighter, and we get osteoporosis. Our blood continues this vicious cycle of stealing calcium from our bones to regulate blood-pH homeostasis. Another problem with a high-animal-protein diet is over-production of uric acid, which crystallizes in our blood. Crystallized uric acid gets trapped in joints and our big toe, causing arthritis and gout! Do you have gout or arthritis? Gout is an overproduction of uric acid due to a high-animal-protein diet. Both of these conditions are very painful and debilitating.

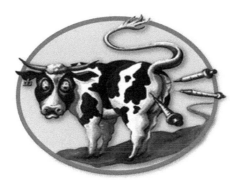

80% of all U.S. Antibiotics are Given to Cows.

Dairy Products ARE the MOST recalled products by the FDA.

Containing the following:

Contaminates	Staphylococci
Listeria	Mycobacterium
Deadly E. Coli	Paratuberculosis
Hormoes	Antibiotics
GMOs	Cortigol- Stress

Why take the RISK!

Kidney stones are calcium from our bones!

Animal Protein Makes Us a BITCH!

A high-protein, animal-based diet which includes meat, cheese, chicken, seafood, and saturated fats, causes dangerous side effects in the human body. ***Don't be fooled by the ketogenic diet!*** Nobody will argue that the ketogenic diet has the capability to create dramatic weight loss. The real question is: Dramatic weight loss at what cost? There is overwhelming evidence that a diet high in animal products will cause premature death. The ketogenic diet opens wide the door for a vascular or malignant event that will result in premature death, dementia, and a miserable life. Is it worth taking that risk? You can achieve weight loss on a whole-food, plant-based diet that eliminates chronic disease, inflammation, and vascular risk, and markedly reduces the risk from all cancers. Simply put: The ketogenic diet will result in premature death. The only difference will be in what size of casket you will be buried in.

Facts make me CRY!! The following is a short list of the dangerous components and health hazards in animal products:

B: Bacterial Protein Toxins (BPT)

I: Insulin Growth Factor-1 (IGF-1)

T: TMOA, trimethylamine oxide

C: Cholesterol from animals in EXCESS

H: Heart Disease and Hypertension

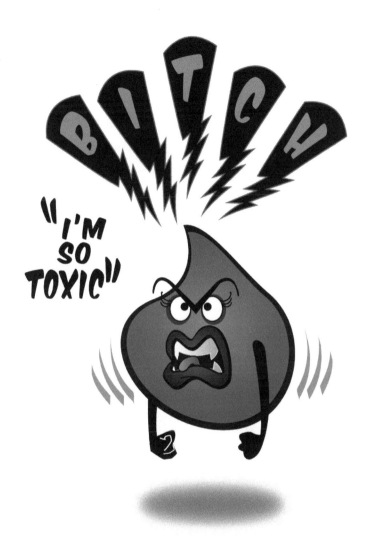

Bacterial Protein Toxins*:* BPT is in the muscles and breast milk of all living creatures, including humans. After the purest of organic animal products are ingested, BPT causes immediate inflammation and stiffening of blood vessels, which is endotoxemia. It takes hours to "flush our blood" of bacterial protein toxins! Examples of a BPT breakfast are: Bacon, eggs, butter, sausage, cottage cheese, yogurt, etc. This vicious cycle depletes the immune system. No matter how you "pre-treat" animal products, ***bacterial protein toxins*** (BPT) are *stable and cannot* be destroyed by cooking, boiling, or baking, and they cannot be dissolved in our stomach acids. BPT creates acute and constant inflammation, which results in chronic disease. BPT attacks the endothelial cells, which line our blood vessels. Endothelial cells relax and constrict our blood vessels autonomically. These important muscular cells become damaged and stiff. This is the beginning of atherosclerosis, hardening of our arteries.

Insulin Growth Factor-1 (IGF-1) is also present in *all* living creatures. IGF-1 is the single most powerful hormone that promotes the *growth* of anything. When we consume IGF-1 from beef and dairy products, however, it *opens* the doors to bad genes, thereby putting us at risk for cancer. According to the China Study, IGF-1 is designed to do a job: To seek opportunities to grow "anything!" According to the China Study:

> *"IGF-1 is the number one cancer-hormone*
> *involved in cancer growth,*
> *cancer promotion in every stage of cancer,*
> *including spread and invasion."*

Babies and teenagers naturally have higher levels of IGF-1 in their blood because they are growing. Human breast milk provides IGF-1 to help a newborn grow from seven to 15 pounds. The breast milk of a cow helps a calf grow from 90 to 900 pounds. However, we do *not* want IGF-1 from a cow. Higher levels of IGF-1 beyond early childhood and puberty are dangerous for adults! IGF-1 from beef and dairy products is the number-one cancer-promoting, growth-promoting hormone *committed* to *every* stage of cancer, which is growth, spread, and invasion. If you have cancer or had cancer, do not consume *any* dairy products, including nonfat yogurt. Nonfat yogurt has higher concentrations of IGF-1 because the fat is removed, and the IGF-1 is concentrated. In addition, estrogen in beef and chicken is just like human estrogen. Our body treats it as its own and increases abnormal cell production. The occurrences of breast cancer in women and prostate cancer in men increase with the regular consumption of animal products.

Trimethylamine Oxide (TMAO) is converted from lecithin, which is found only in animal foods. During digestion, the gut microbiome converts lecithin into TMAO, causing severe inflammation inside our blood vessels. Gut microbiome comprises trillions and trillions of bacteria that function in the large intestines. Gut microbiome is CREATED from the food we eat, and it can ruin our lives! TMAO makes the insides of our arteries rough and jagged, allowing animal cholesterol to stick to the arterial walls of our blood vessels. This is the beginning of atherosclerotic plaque formation, which narrows blood vessels, causing high blood pressure, which is the cause of strokes and heart attacks.

Atherosclerosis begins in high school and continues in our twenties. It does not matter how strong, athletic, young, or thin you are. Thin, young, athletic people can have diabetes, high cholesterol, and high blood pressure. During the Korean War, the bodies of young soldiers, killed in combat, were returned to the United States. During autopsy, 80 percent of these 20-year-old soldiers already had atherosclerotic plaques in their blood vessels. These young, fit U.S. soldiers already had atherosclerosis by their late teens. The foundation was set for a future stroke or heart attack.

Finally, the World Health Organization classified processed meats such as bacon, sausage, hot dogs, and ham as a Group I Carcinogen. It's time to walk away from the Standard American Diet.

Cholesterol, made by our bodies, is needed for healthy hormone production. Animal cholesterol is the extra cholesterol that we store as body fat and which causes circulatory damage! Animal cholesterol does the following:

- It collects in our breasts, abdomen, and vital organs.

- It becomes fat storage throughout the body and arteries.

- It clogs *all* arteries, causing a stroke and/or heart attack.

- It blocks *insulin* from getting glucose into muscle and brain cells

- It causes Diabetes-2, decreasing our energy and focus!

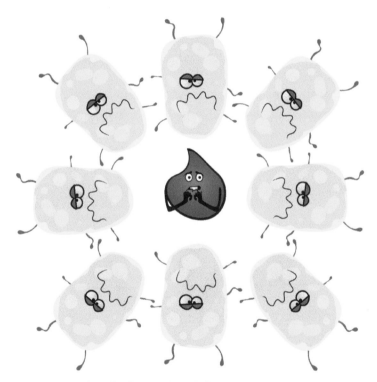

OUR BODY HAS AN UNLIMITED CAPACITY TO STORE FAT IN THE ABDOMEN & LIVER CAUSING FATTY LIVER DISEASE.

Heart disease is the number-one killer of all humans

Seventeen million people die worldwide from heart attacks each year. High blood pressure, the silent killer, is present for years before a stroke and/or a heart attack occurs. Studies reveal that being on blood pressure medications does not lengthen life. Salt is the biggest culprit to high blood pressure! We need a minimum of 400 mg of sodium per day. However, with the Standard American Diet, coupled with processed foods and dining out, we consume more than 4,000 mg of salt per day. This is 10-fold of the amount that we need. Too much salt is addictive and toxic to the body.

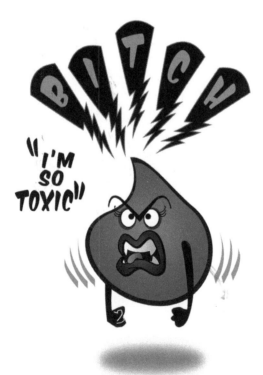

When we eat an animal-based diet too high in toxic proteins, our life becomes a BITCH. We become DIABOLICAL…

D: Diabetes-2

I: Ischemia

A: Alzheimer's

B: Brain Fog

O: Overweight

L: Lethargic

I: Irritable

C: Cancer Opportunities

A: Autoimmune Disorders

L: Liver is Fatty

Yes, I was a *diabolical bitch.* There is no way around this reality. Meat and cheese damage us beyond our worst nightmares. We run out of energy and become frustrated regularly because of our daily dose of toxins. *We deserve better.* When I discovered how metabolic syndrome was destroying the quality of my life through my own doing, I had to *pause.* Was it worth eating all the *bacon* I wanted as my lovely world crumbled around me? No. So I took a stand. Forget about ALL the reasons *you should give up* excess proteins. Right now, give yourself one reason why you deserve better health. All you need is ***one reason***. More than anything... Do it for you! If you want to reduce personal suffering on many levels, give up meat and cheese. Doing so is a game-changer.

7. Complex Carbohydrates to the Rescue!

O ur last chapter covered a lot of bad news about animal-based proteins. Clearly, we have a lot to lose by following a high-animal-protein diet. Our goal is to avoid, stop, and reverse metabolic syndrome, the gateway to chronic disease.... Now for the good news!

What is an Anti-Inflammatory Diet?

An anti-inflammatory diet *is not* the Standard American Diet, but a diet rich in whole complex carbohydrates such as grains, beans, vegetables, fruits, and a few nuts. Plants are anti-inflammatory. When our diet comprises 50 percent of whole grains, beans, and starchy vegetables, and 50 percent of fruits and non-starchy vegetables, we obtain all the calories, proteins, nutrients, and energy that we need!

Now, wait a minute! We are bacon lovers, but we are supposed to live on *plants* alone? That sounds dreadful! But hang in there with me. In just two weeks on a plant-based diet, you will discover surprises, benefits, and new experiences from eating creative, delicious, and filling plant-based dishes. Your taste buds will change, your health will improve, and your energy level will soar! When you understand the consequences of what you eat, you will not look back on the Standard American Diet. Take the plunge!

Grains & Beans (50%)
Vegetables & Fruit (50%)

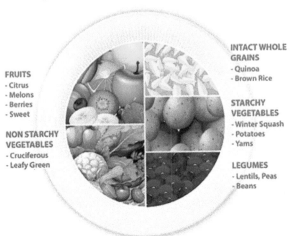

FRUITS
- Citrus
- Melons
- Berries
- Sweet

NON STARCHY VEGETABLES
- Cruciferous
- Leafy Green

INTACT WHOLE GRAINS
- Quinoa
- Brown Rice

STARCHY VEGETABLES
- Winter Squash
- Potatoes
- Yams

LEGUMES
- Lentils, Peas
- Beans

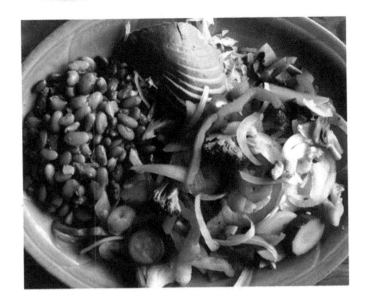

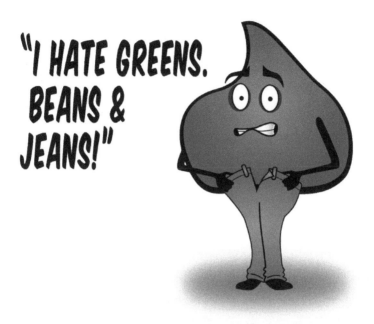

"I HATE GREENS, BEANS & JEANS!"

It is that simple. The concept of "incomplete proteins" was debunked years ago. Remember, the *liver* is your LIBRARY of recycled amino acids, available as needed. Your liver makes thousands of proteins just for your body's needs! One of the few recommended supplements is Vitamin B-12. *B is for Bacteria*! A plant-based diet heals immediately, and chronic disease reverses.

However, be careful! Processed plant-foods and vegetable *oils* are extremely high in calories and are not necessary! Just like cows, we manufacture our own cholesterol, which is needed for normal hormone function. I have been oil-free for four years, and there is nothing fat-free about me. Highly processed plants in such forms as bread, veggie burgers, and vegan protein bars contain less *fiber*, minerals, and vitamins. Soy protein-isolates, found in many processed vegan foods, promote cancer growth. In addition, extra salt, oil, and sugar make these foods high in calories. Avoid them.

Meet the Stomach… Wait for it!

When do we stop eating: (1) When we are full? or (2) When we have had enough calories? We stop eating when our stomachs are *full*. Our stomach is a muscular hollow folded sac, tucked under our ribs. When we completely fill up, this sac is about half a gallon! Sure, stomach sizes vary based on body size, hormones, eating patterns, and muscle contractions. We stop eating when our half-gallon tank is full, no matter what we put into it: Broccoli or cheesecake! It takes 15 minutes for our stomach's stretch receptors to signal our brain to stop eating. Those last 15 minutes get us into trouble…Right? *Pause* before you are stuffed because there's no such thing as *moderation*! Be mindful, thoroughly chew your food, and put your fork down between bites. RELAX. Our goal is to establish a pattern of healthy eating over a lifetime. Instead of eating a high-calorie, zero-fiber meal of oils, meat, and cheese, eat a bulky meal high in plants, fiber, nutrients, and low in calories that requires a *pause before you are full*. Breathe, *wait for it,* and be patient. Do not drink any fluids during meals because they cause bloating and indigestion. Let the stomach acids digest food in your stomach. Excess fluids rush undigested food into the small intestines. You can drink water two hours after a meal.

Four-hundred calories of broccoli and potatoes equal the volume of our stomach, approximately a half-gallon. Plants do not have harmful byproducts, hormones, and toxins like animal protein. Four-hundred calories comprise two tablespoons of oil, which leaves our stomach empty and hungry! *Oil* is dense in calories. Completely avoid it! A calorie is a unit of energy that fuels normal bodily function, brain energy, and muscle activity. Not all calories are equal because foods have different calorie densities. A gram of *fat* is nine calories, while a gram of protein or carbohydrate is only four calories. Alcohol is seven calories a gram. Make complex carbohydrates, whole plants, your dietary mainstay. You will lose weight!

The biggest surprise I found in changing to a whole-food, plant-based diet was the volume of food I could eat at one meal. Suddenly, I had to schedule time around meals in order to *chew* my food and RELAX! Initially you might experience some discomfort from your stomach's stretch receptors. But take a gentle walk and continue with your busy day. Soon, your blood glucose levels will rise as you get three to five hours of focused energy to complete your tasks.

Sometimes, I felt like a boa constrictor that had consumed an enormous meal. *Pause* and say your prayers of gratitude. Something amazing happens: Energy and blood glucose levels after the consumption of a whole-food, plant-based meal steadily rise for hours! At times, six hours would pass, and I would completely forget to eat. Complex carbohydrates give you plenty of protein without the added cholesterol, toxins, or calories.

Complex Carbohydrate and Diabetes-2

Complex carbohydrates are *plants*! They are fruits, vegetables, nuts, beans, and grains. Complex carbohydrates are "sugars linked together." The *only* nutrient the brain and muscles can use is *glucose,* which is the most important carbohydrate. Glucose is transported into the brain and muscle cells by *insulin.* Diabetes-2 develops when animal cholesterol acts like cellophane wrap and *blocks* insulin from getting glucose into cells. However, when we don't have excess fat circulating through our blood, glucose from plants is slowly released into the bloodstream, giving us a continuous infusion of clean energy. You will experience focused energy for hours to do your jobs, and solve problems. Plants are the cleanest *fuel* for humans. It's like driving a solar-powered Tesla versus a diesel truck.

When we eat too many whole plants, excess glucose is stored as glycogen in the liver, blood, and muscles until it is needed; that's about two tablespoons. Using up this reserve glycogen is equivalent to running full speed for an hour! Then, you're completely out of energy. Glucagon is the hormone that converts glycogen back to glucose for immediate energy.

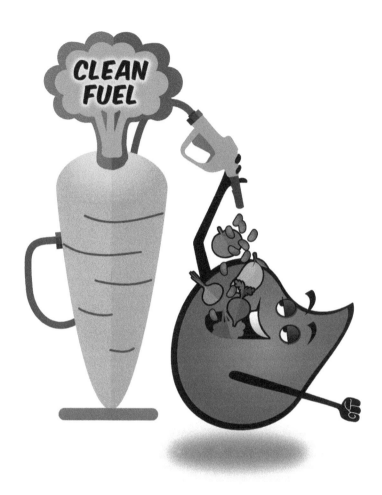

What's Fiber Got to Do with It?

When I was a colonoscopy nurse, I could dress a man in three minutes flat, regardless of his size, age, or frailty. After a colonoscopy, patients would be sedated with versed and fentanyl. This would make patients relaxed, forgetful, and very talkative. Without my patients knowing, I would assemble their clothes in order of shoes, socks, underwear, loose-fitting pants, belt, undershirt, button-down shirt, and jacket. When they stood up, all items of clothing would miraculously be maneuvered up their bodies without them knowing. Patients would say, "How did you do that?" Because patients were under the influence of powerful but short-acting drugs, much of what I said was forgotten. However, patients were always sent home with colorful photos of their colons, typed instructions, and hand-written instructions about *fiber*. Why is fiber so important in preventing colon cancer?

Fiber promotes intestinal health. It is like a rough washcloth that scrubs the insides of both our large and small intestines. Fiber grabs excess cholesterol, extra hormones, dense processed debris, and toxins from the walls of the colon and escorts them out of the body as fecal waste through the rectum. Hurray for fiber! Without fiber, toxins linger in the large colon causing constipation. The longer toxins stay in the large colon, the more likely they will irritate the colon wall, creating polyps. Polyps, over time, can become a source of cancer growth. Fiber is present *only* in plants, not in animal products; and fiber keeps us fuller for longer, and traps nutrients in the small intestine for *slower* digestion. Therefore, glucose from complex carbohydrates enters the bloodstream at a *slower* pace, which also helps us lose weight!

Research on *microbiome, which is bacteria from food,* is exploding! The microbiome's favorite meal is the byproducts of digested fiber which is from plants, the main ingredient of *beneficial gut* bacteria. You don't need expensive probiotics. If you are on a whole-food, plant-based diet, you will *not* have constipation. The average American gets under 10 grams of fiber per day. Humans need 25 to 35 grams of fiber per day. However meat, fish, eggs, and dairy products contain *NO* fiber.

CANCER KILLING CELLS-
YOUR NEW BEST FRIEND!

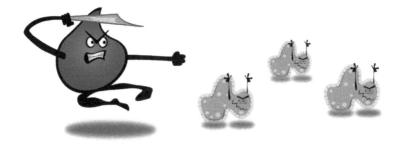

Binding Protein Levels: Your New Best Friend!

Eating more plants increases protein binding levels in your body. Remember, any animal protein is harmful to you. But you *cannot* get too much protein on a whole-food, plant-based diet! Your body works hard to eradicate abnormal cells that contribute to cancer growth. These cells are called cancer-killing cells and binding protein levels which create a *hostile* environment for *all* cancers! This is great news and one of my favorite reasons for giving up meat and cheese for a *diet rich* in green *warriors* that aggressively snuff out cancer cells.

In fact, the blood of a plant-based individual is eight times more likely to snuff out cancer cells than the blood of a dairy- and meat-eating carnivore. The hormone IGF-1 circulating in the blood, from dairy and beef, feeds new cancer cells! *I'm sold on the vegan diet!*

8. Rage and the Power of You!

For me, making the decision to give up animal products, salt, oil, and sugar was devastating! It was like saying goodbye to my best friend. No more salmon, cheese, bacon and eggs. How my tears flowed! However, the science behind the whole-food, plant-based diet was overwhelming, and my healing began in days. Personal suffering downsized, and so did my body! A simmering fury crept over me. Why was this easy fix hidden from me and from millions of other suffering Americans? How much time did I lose? How many opportunities came and went because I was too sick and anxious to do anything, too confused?

Emotion is energy in motion. This newfound experience is willpower and motivation, which allows you to do radical, inconvenient tasks, such as changing your food choices! Can you remember a time in your life when you carried out a herculean event or solo project against all the odds? Why did you do it? What kept you going? How committed are you to the outcome of learning a new skill or acquiring a new possession? Knowledge is the key to end needless suffering across the globe! We are all connected. A simple change in diet allows you to gain more than you can imagine.

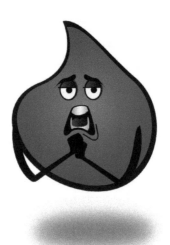

"I'M BEGGING YOU - GIVE UP MEAT & CHEESE! DO IT FOR ME. DO IT FOR US. I LOVE YOU!"

<u>*Who's Behind All This Suffering?*</u>

I love the Blame Game, but it's dangerous! If someone else is to blame, then responsibility for change and healing does not lie within you. Blaming others prevents us from making real change. Be informed, empowered, and committed to new and delicious foods. What I discovered in the industries of healthcare, pharmaceuticals, and factory farming, and in the beef and dairy lobbies, is... *everyone is suffering* and dying from premature, preventable chronic diseases.

Less than 2 percent of the U.S, population is whole-food plant-based!

Consuming animal and seafood products damages our micro-blood circulation system with excess cholesterol, which goes everywhere in our bodies! Our blood doesn't know what to do with the excess cholesterol. These toxins end up in tiny places, like our eyes, ears, big toes, brain, lungs, heart, and liver. We become hard of hearing, our vision diminishes, we get confused, we become pre-diabetic, we contract heart disease and arthritis, gout plagues our big toe, and we have difficulty breathing. Our liver loses the battle of cleaning and filtering our blood. Large, fatty deposits from excess cholesterol appear in our liver!

Over time, fatty liver disease becomes part of metabolic syndrome from the cholesterol we eat. Common bloodwork reveals abnormal, elevated liver enzymes that are double normal values. Patients are often screened for hepatitis B, C, and other treatable causes of chronic liver disease. A scheduled abdominal ultrasound reveals a *fatty, enlarged liver which is hepatomegaly.* Our beloved patient is diagnosed with non-alcohol fatty liver disease (NAFLD) . In 1988, the incidence of NAFLD was about 5 percent of the population. Today, it is a staggering 25 to 30 percent of the U.S. population. That is a 500-percent increase! Today, 70 million to 100 million Americans have a spectrum of fatty liver disease directly linked to the American Standard Diet, **SAD**.

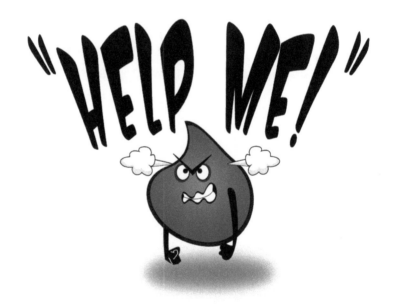

NAFLD is the number-one cause
of liver abnormalities in the United States,
costing $300 billion annually!

How difficult is it to get a healthy, available liver? Almost impossible!! Twenty years ago, the biggest healthcare epidemic was Hepatitis C, which affected four million Americans! Currently, Hepatitis C is readily treated by newly developed drugs. However, NAFLD, a food disease, will become the number-one reason for liver transplants because it leads to liver cancer!

Who wants to be waiting for a new Liver, all for the love of cheese and meat?

NAFLD impacts 70 million to 100 million Americans because of our food choices of meat, cheese and seafood. However, we can enjoy delicious foods that taste like meat and cheese which are *not animal-based and harmful*. Fatty liver disease is worth avoiding at all costs. The personal suffering, expense, and loss of quality of life are provocative and overreaching.

The American healthcare system is the best in the world when it comes to diagnosis and treatment. However, it fails miserably at prevention and addressing the root cause of chronic disease. U.S. healthcare providers and medical students get minimal education on nutrition and how food relates to chronic disease. Most nutrition classes taught at universities *today* are based on incorrect information!

Big Pharma influences the academic focus of many medical schools in favor of drug treatment as opposed to prevention. Medical students spend hundreds of hours studying organic and bio-chemistry and pharmaceutical agents, but typically receive few hours in nutrition. Ask most doctors what your food has to do with your diagnosis, and most would say, "Nothing, or very little impact." Corporate medical practices allow 15 to 20 minutes per patient visit, which allows just enough time to make a diagnosis and write a prescription. In addition, many doctors receive 100 emails per day from their other patients. Healthcare providers are *"the blind leading the blind."* If your doctor isn't asking about your diet, he or she is doing you a grave disservice.

Western medicine and Big Pharma have failed us at a fundamental level. As we get sick, we are robbed of our mind, our decision-making, our body, and our dignity. Every penny and ounce of freedom are taken, and we declare, *"This is not my fault."* It's time to wake up, look around, and *stop* this trend. You deserve better.

Is it radical and unfair to give up meat and cheese? Maybe. Is it radical and unfair to attend a funeral for a 50-year-old man who unexpectedly died from liver failure or a heart attack leaving behind a wife and three young children? Is it unfair that 90 percent of heart attack victims will not survive? Yes, it's unfair that you'll spend a significant amount of your income on healthcare expenses, hospitalizations, and prescriptions, leaving little room for vitality, joy, and laughter.

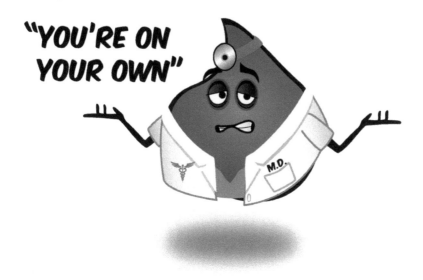

"YOU'RE ON YOUR OWN"

The beef and dairy industries are killing us slowly. Big Pharma and the healthcare industry are cashing in big time! Don't be a part of this vicious, downward spiral. Get out while you can! Now is the time to take in *new* information and change the outcome of your life. Don't be the victim of your uninformed choices! Be the hero and creator of your life, every day, by avoiding meat, cheese, and seafood. Gregg Braden, a famous speaker and scientist exploring quantum physics and behavior change, states that when the facts are clear, the choice is obvious. He continues with this:

> *"When people put together the right information at the right time, and think for themselves, they will make wise choices to thrive, survive and simultaneously build resilience."*

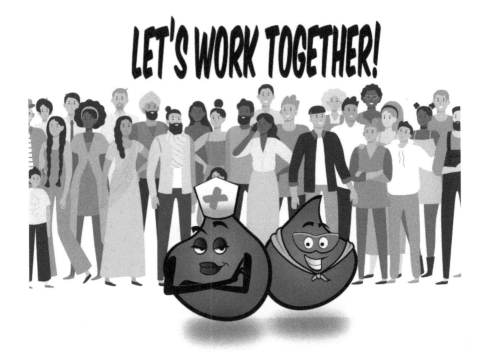

9. The 14-Day Blood Challenge!

T his is the chapter we have been waiting for! The Treatment Plan is the 14-Day *Blood Challenge*! If you want to do this on your own, make it an adventure! You can use existing bloodwork results if you have them or schedule a doctor's visit and get your bloodwork done. All we are tracking are total cholesterol, triglycerides, and blood pressure. For now, forget about the BMI. This number does not change in a two-week period. If you choose to follow the Blood Challenge over one to two months, no worries! However, be specific and stick to the food program. Plan for two large meals per day, at 9 a.m. and 3 p.m., with NO snacks. Your two meals should include:

- Breakfast: 1 cup each: oatmeal, beans, and fruit
- Late Lunch: 1 cup each: grains, beans, and large salad
- Late Lunch: 2 cups of Steamed Vegetables. RELAX.
- Avoid salt, oil, and sugar. Avoid caffeine
- Drink water between meals, NOT during meals.
- Drink 8+ glasses of water per day.

Essentially, this is intermittent fasting. Rest your digestive tract between meals. You can do it. Follow this program on your own, or with a friend. You'll observe your blood values quickly improve at the end of the 14-day challenge. One of my favorite dishes is a whole baked potato, with steamed broccoli, and low-sodium marinara sauce.

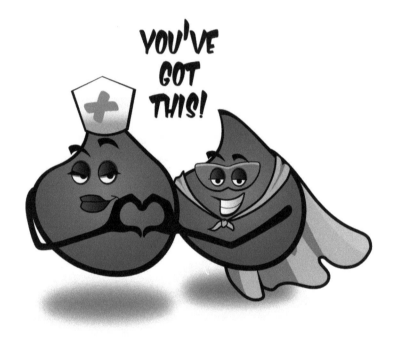

You want to be full after these two large meals. It takes almost an hour to eat because you are slowly chewing high-fiber fruits for breakfast and high-fiber vegetables for lunch. Take a moment to digest your food, walk, and get ready for your afternoon. You are re-programming your body and taste buds back to the original human diet that supports a longer, more productive life. After you eat a whole-food, plant-based meal, sit quietly for about 15 minutes in order for your stomach's stretch receptors to calm down. During this time, complex carbohydrates enter the digestive track, and blood glucose levels begin to rise. Hunger pangs go away, and energy returns to your body and mind. A whole-food, plant-based diet maintains blood glucose levels over a longer period of time, and there are no toxic byproducts from this meal.

On the next page is a very basic food chart. Be sure to record each meal in the chart.

Day / Date	1	2	3	4	5
Breakfast (9 AM)					
Lunch (3 PM)					
Water					
Activities					
Feelings					

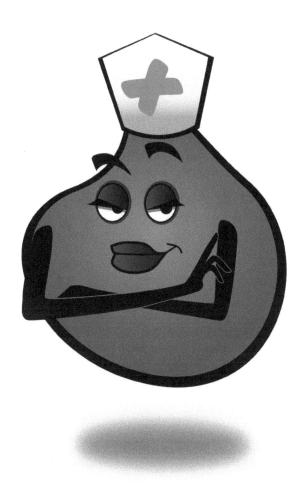

NOTES:

If you already have a recording program that you enjoy, use that program to record your success! Every day record your activities and your feelings. Write down two things you are grateful for. Also, note your desire to be healthy, strong, and free. Take a moment to breathe deeply and sit in silence. Two meals per day is all you need! Have a beautiful feast of steamed vegetables, fresh green salad, baked potato at 3 pm. You'll still be satisfied at 6 pm. Go to bed early and for breakfast, enjoy grains and fresh fruit! Remember, food is our homework, not a trusted friend.

It is okay to miss your old foods! At this point, rename those foods! Remind yourself why you renamed your foods and how animal-based products cause acute inflammation and rob us of precious time and vitality. During this challenge, stick with basic foods, and keep it simple during the challenge! Do something special for yourself, like schedule a massage, take a walk, acupuncture, or visit a friend. Acknowledge your effort and give yourself a hug!

Make sure your kitchen and refrigerator have been cleared of tempting foods like ice cream, cheese, yogurt, and eggs. Tofu and ground flaxseed are fabulous substitutes for eggs, especially when served with steamed spinach and oil-free hash browns. You can do this! It will change your life. Your body will thank you. I remember when I started losing weight, I felt sad to see it go. I made a point of "thanking the weight" and sending it on its way!

The 14-Day Blood Challenge

Don't Skip **Breakfast (8 a.m. or 9 a.m.)**: 1 cup each: beans & oats,

2 cups: Fruit, ½ cup: almond milk, Black Strap Molasses, Flaxseed.

> **You will feel **Full**, chew slowly!

> **Stretch & Walk in the Morning. What are you grateful for?

Drink **Water**: Drink water up to 30 minutes before meals &

> Wait 2 hours after meals. Water with meals cause Indigestion.

Lunch (2 p.m. or 3 p.m.): Large Veggie Salad with cooked vegetables,

> *Beans, and warm grains.

> *Salad Dressing: fresh lemon, tahini, hummus.
> Warm Grains

> *Ex: Baked potato, steamed broccoli with Marinara Sauce.

> *Keep it whole & plant-based: Grains, Beans & Vegetables

Drink Water between Breakfast & Lunch (10 a.m. to 1:30 p.m.)

WALK after Meals: Record your thoughts, wishes, and prayers.

I am **grateful** for #1, #2, #3…

Repeat what you **LOVE**: #1, #2, #3…

Reach out to a friend or family member.

Be caring and Be open!

Evening: 3rd Meal is not necessary! Keep it small: veggies with hummus.

Go to bed early, hungry and plan Breakfast! Warm herbal tea,

Vegetable broth. Calming activities. Deep Breathing and read.

NO: Salt, Oil, Refined sugar, Vinegar, hot-spices, alcohol, caffeine,

Semi-processed foods like toast.

** *FOOD is HOMEWORK, not a Friend or Entertainment*!

10. Ride the Magic Carpet with Me!

We explored life-threatening dangers of consuming the Standard American Diet, <u>SAD</u>. What happens when we chose a plant-based diet? For someone who loves salmon, cheese, bacon and eggs, this better be worth it!

Let's get back to our typical American patient suffering from metabolic syndrome. He has an encyclopedia of symptoms and diagnoses, including fatty liver disease that would make any physician's head spin! All these symptoms are *related* to two problems:

Decrease in Blood Circulation due to excess cholesterol which narrows arteries.
Acute & constant inflammation causing chronic disease.

Our beloved American patient follows the advice of his doctor and takes ten medications as prescribed. In the next twelve months, the FDA will likely approve a billion-dollar new drug for the treatment of fatty liver disease without ever mentioning a food change. Will his poor health be cured by this additional medication? No, these powerful medications have side effects that put us at risk for adverse effects.

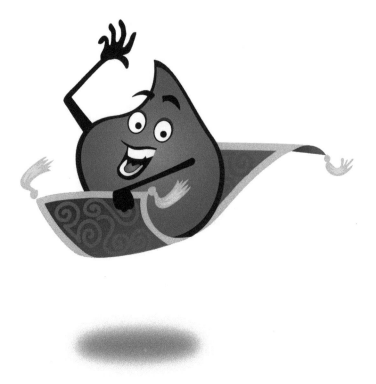

___What Will You Gain by Changing Your Food Choices?___

What if our typical patient chooses a whole food, plant-based diet? The following conditions will be dramatically diminish because:

(1) There's more room in the blood vessels and

(2) Acute inflammation will stop and circulation to the brain, liver, heart, and kidneys improve, along with the following:

- Blood pressure improves

- Diabetes-2 diminishes

- Atherosclerosis improves

- Heart Disease improves

- Sexual Performance Improves

- Brain fog, Confusion & dementia Improves

- Constipation diminishes

- Anxiety & Depression Improves

These are predictable and reproducible results in patients who choose a WFPB diet. Within days, blood pressure begins to drop. Blood vessels heal as the repetitive vascular injury from animal-based toxins is stopped. The lipid profile improves because plants have zero cholesterol. 100 percent of participants in my two-week Blood Challenge Class had improvements in their blood work simply by changing their highly processed diet to a whole food, plant-based diet. Dr. Caldwell Esselstyn's data demonstrates that a WFPB diet halts and reverses atherosclerotic vascular disease. Cardiac patients with narrowing of the coronary arteries improve significantly without the need for expensive, invasive procedures like stenting or coronary artery bypass which is open-heart surgery! The WFPB diet has a thirty-fold better outcome in preventing a second heart attack compared to the best available cardiac procedures.

Evidence shows a WFPB diet improves inflammation in those suffering from inflammatory arthritis. The gut microbiome holds the key to many diseases of chronic inflammation. Extensive research is reveals the connection between gut microbiome and inflammatory bowel disease. Today we know the microbiome of a person on a plant-based diet is distinctly different than the microbiome of a person on the SAD.

Diets high in animal fat promote acid reflux, whereas a plant-based diet eliminates acid reflux symptoms! The SAD causes constipation because animal products do not have fiber. More than 90 percent of *all* Americans lack the daily recommended requirement of 30 grams. Constipation does *not* occur on a plant-based diet.

The blood of a whole food, plant-eating person is a cancer "search-and-destroy" operation that finds and snuffs out pre-cancerous cells before they reproduce and cause serious problems. The blood of a person on a plant-based diet has an eight-fold increase in the power to destroy the cancer cells compared to the blood of a person on SAD.

True healing begins, with weight loss, while existing chronic diseases diminish. Several medications can be reduced or eliminated. Mental clarity and outlook improve, and you will experience less anxiety! Dairy and beef products contain the harmful stress hormone cortisol, which increases anxiety levels. The lives of a cow, a pig, a chicken, and other animals in husbandry are hellacious and terrifying, which increases their cortisol levels! Modern medicine disconnects our symptoms from the root causes of disease. Similarly, we disconnect from the source and conditions of the animals we consume, daily. Watching *Meet, your Meat* was enough for me to be cured from ever eating beef, chicken, or bacon again!

When we give up cholesterol, toxins, and extra hormones, blood circulation improves to our brains; we feel smarter and brighter! We have fewer doctors' appointments, fewer symptoms, and fewer excuses from doing what we really want to do. We have more time and money.

It is very difficult for metabolic syndrome patients to lose weight, unless they begin the whole-food, plant-based diet. Dr. Michael Greger, the author of *How Not to Die*, and his website, www.NutritionFacts.org, is a gift to mankind! Most questions about food are answered on his website. Watch him on YouTube as well. Dr. Greger is an invaluable, entertaining source of information for the metabolic syndrome patient!

One of my favorite ancient texts is the Bhagavad Gita, from India. It is 1,500 years old and is the oldest, longest epic poem known to mankind. It has been turned into a five-hour Hollywood film and a five-day movie in India. Its message is that life is hard, but…

Any action in the right direction is better than NO action at all.

Even with my home burning to the ground in the Santa Rosa Fires of 2017, the quality, calmness, and joy in my life dramatically increased. I felt freedom, abundance, generosity, resilience, and capable of solving life's biggest challenges. I began to meet others who were whole-food, plant-based, and I connected with a beautiful community that was like family. It is a community of smart, forward-thinking people from around the world that cares about others, their communities, and the future of mankind and the environment. We are all connected! The WFPB movement is only 2-percent strong at present, but it's growing every day! I know this book resonates with you, and I wholeheartedly welcome you to this community! You are a part of this wonderful, abundant movement that is changing the world, one person at a time!

It's exciting to teach my class *Truth in Food, the Blood Knows!*, observe the participants, and see, hear, and experience their health improving. Their bloodwork results speak volumes, before and after the 14-Day Blood Challenge!

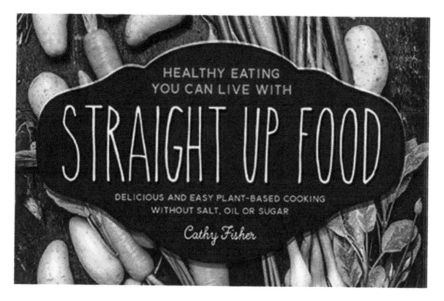

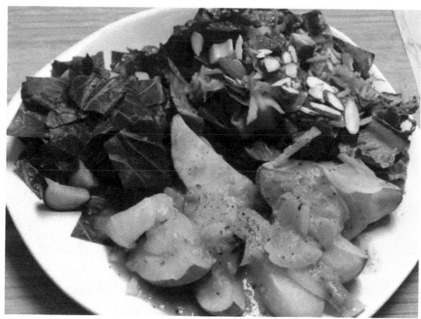

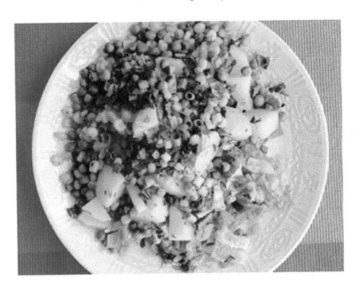

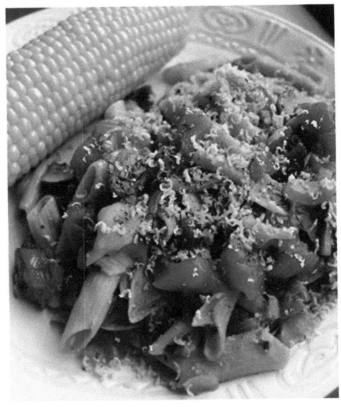

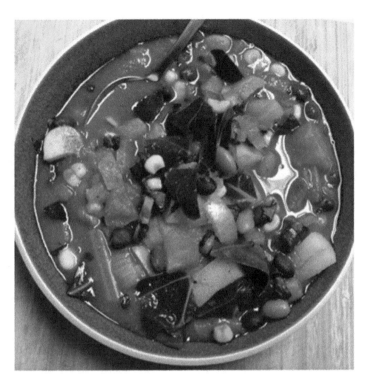

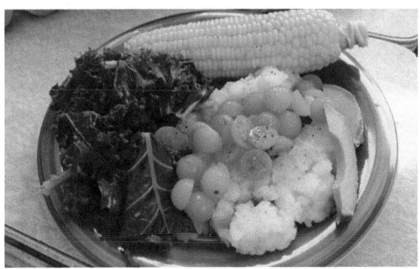

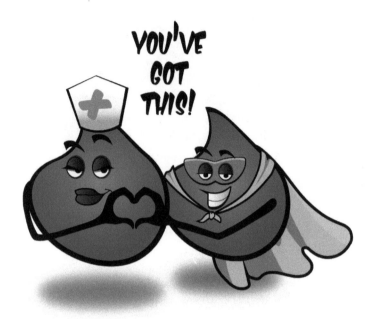

It was a great privilege to teach one of my classes with Cathy Fisher, the famous blogger, and author of *Straight Up Food*. Cathy has more than 20 years of experience in being a whole-food, plant-based chef. She provided insight into some of the obstacles this diet change creates for you:

- It's too hard and time-consuming.

- It's radical, and no one else is doing this!

- I won't like the taste of "this new food."

- I don't want to be the "odd-ball out!"

- It's too expensive!

- I won't be able to dine out anymore.

- What's a good label, and what's a bad label?

- I live with people who don't eat this way.

- How do I start from scratch?

- I'm too busy and stressed!

- Do I have to use your recipes?

- How do I stay compliant?

- How do I add more flavor to the foods?

- How can I possibly find support?

Yes, each of us may have a million reasons not to pursue this lifestyle, but none of them hold water when it comes to the health and life-saving benefits of a plant-based diet. Where do I get my *joy* and *pleasure*? Re-think this concept of joy and pleasure we all deserve. My food is now my homework. When I eat well, my next three to five hours are guaranteed to be productive and focused, and eating well puts me in the driver's seat! My tribe arrived in the way of community groups, meet-ups, and making new friends who appreciate and understand my core values. As I had more "brain space" for independent thought and critical thinking, my future became brighter! Food became my homework, my medicine, and I sought out other means of pleasure, joy, and comfort, such as physical activities, hobbies of learning, community outreach, acupuncture, and meditation.

To move along this journey, think in terms of *WANT versus NEED.* Many years ago, when our oldest son was seven years old, we were on vacation at a seaside Boardwalk. While there, my son grabbed my husband's hand and said, "Dad! Life is terrible!" Instantly, he got the attention of both of us.

"What's the problem?" my husband responded.

After finishing a delicious dinner, playing in the sand for the day, and walking along the boardwalk, our son stated, "I have everything I need, but *nothing* I want."

I'll never forget that moment; it could have been a passage from Ecclesiastes. So often what we want, we don't need. In fact, much of what we want is not helpful or good for us! When we separate our needs from our wants, however, we make better choices. Salt, oil, and sugar keep us prisoners.

In concert with your decision to eat differently, plan out your meals and snacks strategically. Anywhere you go, there are grains, beans, and vegetables. Consuming dairy and beef will always hurt you and ultimately cause early death. Make it a rule: It's not an option.

Making this food change *is* challenging because we're only 2-percent strong. Find your tribe; they're waiting for you! Do not be surprised if you get ridiculed by family members and close friends about going plant-based. Be ready for the typical question: "Where do you get your protein?" Or, "How can you have strong bones without dairy?" Armed with real knowledge, you will respond with, "Where do you get your information?" Reach out to local and national plant-based support groups and resources, including:

- Vegan Meetup Groups
- PCRM (Physicians' Committee for Responsible Medicine)
- NutritionFacts.org
- Cooking classes at junior colleges
- Food for Life classes
- Online cooking demonstrations

Everywhere I go, everyone is curious about this plant-based diet movement! No one belittles me. Forbes Magazine stated, "2019 is the year of the Vegan." NOW is the time to get on board and be a part of the change that is critically needed in order to reverse your metabolic syndrome and improve your health and the environment at the same time!

When you choose to stop eating meat and cheese, you become part of a bigger solution investing in your future and the future of generations to come. Your life continues to change in beautiful ways. You have a stronger, cleaner blood circulation that protects your big and small organs for a better quality of life! Your mind and brain provide top-quality service to your daily needs and challenges. Health is happiness! You've got this!

Sadly, the uninformed person will wait until there is an adverse life event such as a diagnosis of cancer, stroke, heart attack, kidney failure, cirrhosis, etc., before considering a change. This person will know, intuitively, "Something's not right, but I don't know what it is. Who am I to believe?" Believe your blood because it is fighting for your life every day. Give your blood what it needs to survive and thrive: A whole-food, plant-based diet.

Five years ago, I was in a very dark place in my life. I felt terrible, and I was only 40! Symptoms such as brain fog, hypoglycemia, fatigue, anger, depression, and sleep apnea robbed me of the joys in my life, and I was at a complete loss as to what to do. I was too young to feel so poorly. Metabolic syndrome robbed me of the life I deserved. Not satisfied with an early death sentence, I searched the world for real solutions. My mother, Mary Rose Bacon, was diagnosed with Alzheimer's Disease in her early fifties and suffered a miserable, extended death. Clearly, I was following her footsteps. We were the same in every way. She shared her knowledge with me on the latest vitamins and foods that were "good for you." Little did she know that her information was wrong; she was hoodwinked! We deserve the correct information! Know the rules of survival, and thrive during these extreme and uncertain times.

What we eat matters. It matters to our bodies and to the environment. The animals that we eat are, ultimately, killing us! This is a shout-out to the 70 million to 100 million Americans suffering from metabolic syndrome, the gateway to chronic disease: Take action and change your path. Reverse the damage done by an inflammatory, animal-based diet. You deserve this!

Know the truth and *Rename* your food. No one puts *cyanide* in their mouths because they like how it tastes, creating needless suffering and early death. We need more than the existing medical system of diagnoses and more pills! These statistics give us hope for positive change:

- Most deaths are due to chronic disease, from food.

- Almost 90 percent of diabetes-2 is preventable.

- 80 to 90 percent of heart disease is preventable.

- 40 to 70 percent of cancers are avoidable.

The power is in your hands by choosing a plant-based diet. Break the chain of chronic disease and change the path of your life for good. If everyone ate a plant-based diet, there could be Medicare for *all*!

If you are still skeptical, follow my 14-Day Blood Challenge! You can do this anywhere! Let the changes in your blood convince you of the power food has on your biochemistry … your body! Bloodwork is a fasting lipid panel that can be done anywhere. For 14 days, eat a WFPB diet, then repeat the bloodwork. *Be surprised!*

With the significant changes you will see in just two weeks, imagine the healing that will occur in 90 days to six months to one year on this basic food change. Sure, you may be skeptical, but would you argue with your blood? Would you argue with the cardiologist, nephrologist, or physician who's giving you your next prescription for your newest diagnosis or surgery? You can do it!

Become a champion for the movement of better health and a better environment. And be a champion for yourself! This simple change in diet will change the course of nature, your future, and the future of all those around us, one person at a time. Let your transition to healing, wellness, reversing chronic disease, and weight loss speak volumes to those around you, and get back the life you deserve!

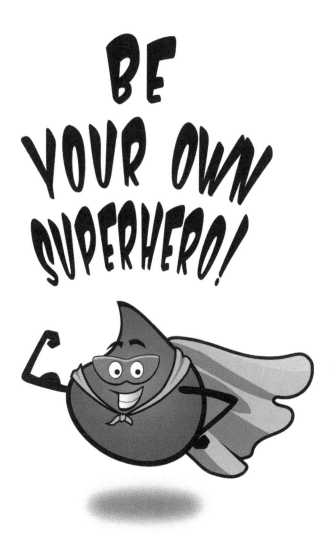

Mary Kay Matossian

References

1. The NEWSTART Program, Weimar, California.

2. PCRM: Physicians Committee of Responsible Medicine, Washington, D.C.

3. The True North Clinic, Santa Rosa, California.

4. Campbell, TC (2006), *THE CHINA STUDY*: United States: First Benbella Books.

5. Campbell, TC (2013), *WHOLE*: Dallas, TX: Benbella Books.

6. Greger, M (2015), *How Not to Die*: NY, NY: Flatiron Books.

7. Barnard, ND (2011), *21 Day Weight Loss Kickstart*: NY, NY: Hachette Book Group.

8. Fuhrman, J (2011), *EAT TO LIVE*: NY, NY: Hachette Book Group.

9. Barnard, ND (2018), *The Vegan Starter Kit*: NY, NY: Hachette Book Group.

10. McDougall, JA (2012), *The Starch Solution*: NY, NY: Rodale Books.

11. Barnard, ND (2017), *The Cheese Trap*: NY, NY: Hachette Book Group.

12. Ornish, D (2019), *UNDO IT!*: NY, NY: Ballantine Books.

13. Campbell, TC (2014), *The LOW-CARB FRAUD*: Dallas, TX: Benbella Books.

14. Barnard, ND (2017), *Reversing Diabetes*: United States: Rodale, Inc.

15. Robbins, J and Robbins, O (2001), *The Food Revolution*.

16. Fisher, C (2016), STRAIGHT UP FOOD: Santa Rosa, CA: Greenbite Publishing.

Documentaries

Forks over Knives

What the Health

Fat, Sick and Nearly Dead

PlantPure Nation

CODE BLUE

GameChanger

Mary Kay Matossian

Acknowledgements

After a four-day visit at the True North Clinic, in Santa Rosa, October of 2016, I became whole-food, plant-based overnight, and never looked back. My healing was so dramatic that it sparked an intense curiosity into the Plants' Movement and Lifestyle. Dr. John McDougall's classes, in Santa Rosa, were informative and entertaining, and always provided buffets of delicious, whole-plant dishes! Dr. McDougall's Advanced Nutrition Weekend, Intensive Medical Workshops, and online course, "The Starch Solution," helped me understand how important food is. I am grateful to the current pioneers of this food and social movement that needs a little push! We are 2-percent strong and growing!

When the veil of poor nutrition was lifted from my eyes, courses, lectures, potlucks, friendships, and communities from around the country emerged, showing me the way to a healthier, happier life. I am grateful!

Thank you, Angela Glasser, for teaching *Ditch the Dairy* and *Whole Plants' Nutrition* at Santa Rosa Junior College. I took Angela's class several times, and she finally asked, "Why do you keep taking my class? It's the same class!" We became fast friends, and she generously shared her knowledge of WFPB cooking. With my nursing background in biometrics, Angela encouraged me to formulate the class, "Truth in Food, the Blood Knows!" A monthly WFPB potluck group was formed that tested my knowledge and skill. All I could bring was fresh fruit! Many of the participants are amazing chefs and share their knowledge with the world, including Cathy Fisher, author of *Straight Up Food* and Katie Mae of TheCulinaryGym.com

After meeting many amazing people within the plants' community, I learned as much as I could. I am grateful to the pioneers who continue to educate the masses, upstream. Dr. Michael Greger's book *How Not to Die* continues to touch millions of lives. His website, www.NutritionFacts.com, is a priceless resource!

The author of The China Study, Dr. Colin Campbell, and his son, Nelson Campbell, Director of Plant Pure Nation, founded the nonprofit Plant Pure Communities called PODS. There are more than 500 Pods in the United States, with a total of more than 170,000 members! There is a POD wherever you go! People are plant-curious, and want to know the truth about food and live a healthier, better life. This is the people's movement, our movement! Everyone is welcome to participate in a brighter, more compassionate future for all.

The PCRM, the Physicians' Committee of Responsible Medicine, successfully sued the FDA for dispensing false information about the "health benefits" of dairy and beef. I'm pleased to be a Food for Life Instructor through the PCRM organization. Food for Life Instructors have access to teach a variety of WFPB classes focusing on the prevention of chronic disease, cancer, and diabetes through cooking demonstrations and educational videos. Thank you for this priceless tool for educating plant-curious participants.

My husband, Harry Berj Matossian, has been especially supportive and a driving force behind my curiosity to live my best life *forward*! As we unearthed these data together on how to reduce chronic disease, he encouraged and continues to encourage me to share this great message of healing!

Thank you for taking the time and reading this book *I Love BACON But…I Love Me More!*

It is women who change the world! One bite at a time! You can make a difference. P.S., No one wants to make this food change, but the outcome and rewards are undeniable! In our lives, in our relationships, and in our coping skills, we're creating happier, healthier families, individuals, and communities all over the globe. Be a part of the Solution!

If you believe in and make these basic food changes, a whole new world of opportunity, love, improved health, and strength will emerge in you and around you! As you change your food, you will feel the difference all the way to the cellular level.

As a gift for your time and consideration, here's a Podcast of the important principles of my book and a short cooking lesson called, "The Thanksgiving Celebration Dish!" See you on the adventure … of *life*!

http://traffic.libsyn.com/tonynavarrasow/MaryMatossianEpisode7Complete.mp3

https://youtu.be/shyGJ67tfiA

www.thebloodchallenge.com

Glossary of Terms

Antioxidants: Substances that reduce damage to the body due to oxygen such as free radicals. Fruits, vegetables, and legumes possess antioxidants which slow the process of aging.

Bloating: Refers to excess "gas" and pressure in the intestinal tract. The two main sources are swallowing air and incomplete digestion of food or excess sugar in the diet. Bloating is caused by dairy, artificial sweeteners, diet soda, chewing gum and drinking excess fluids during a meal.

Calcium: A mineral found in soil which is absorbed into plants with water. A diet high in plants guarantees calcium absorption for healthy bones.

Cholesterol: A waxy, fatty substance produced by living creatures through the liver. It's vital for hormone function, Vitamin D, and cell membrane. Cholesterol consumed from other creatures causes damage and clogs arteries.

Coconut Oil: It is 90% poly-saturated fat which causes dangerously high levels of Low-Density Lipids. This Lousy cholesterol increases the risk of heart disease!

Constipation: Defined as less than 2 bowel movements per week, OR the passage of hard stool requiring straining. Common causes are lack of adequate water, lack of fiber and a diet high in salt, oil and sugar.

Cortisol: The body's main stress hormone which fuels the energy necessary for "Flight or Flight" instinct in a daily crisis which is chronic stress. This hormone plays a role in blood pressure, blood sugar, sleep wake cycle, inflammation and how the body uses carbohydrates, protein, and fats.

DHEA: Dehydroepiandrosterone is a critical, precursor hormone, stored in the body, that converts other hormones into testosterone and estradiol.

Dopamine: A neurotransmitter which sends messages between nerve cells. This is the "Feel Good" neurotransmitter.

Endorphins: This is a group of hormones, secreted within the brain and nervous system that acts our body's natural pain killer. They create feelings of general well-being.

FAT: A compilation of cholesterol, triglycerides and fatty acids which is used for fuel. It is the main source of stored energy and precursors to hormones.

GERD: Gastro Esophageal Reflux Disease occurs when fluid from the stomach leaks into the upper Esophagus which is between the mouth and stomach. The Esophagus becomes irritated. The most common cause is due to obesity and a resultant dysfunctional valve between the Esophagus and the Stomach.

GMO: Genetically Modified Organisms such as corn, wheat, oats, and any plant that has its main DNA modified.

Iodine: An essential mineral used by Thyroid hormones to control metabolism, growth, and repair damaged cells. Seaweed is an excellent source of iodine.

Nutritional Yeast: A good source of B Vitamins and protein.

Oxytocin: A hormone which is released when couples snuggle or bond socially.

Palm Oil: It is a saturated oil which is very high in poly-saturated fat and increases our lousy cholesterol, Low-Density Lipids.

Protein: A Combination of Amino Acids linked together which play a critical role in the structure, function and regulation of muscle cells, body tissues and organs.

Seitan: A protein derived from wheat gluten which is high in protein, low in calories, and contains calcium, iron, potassium and vitamin B.

Serotonin: A hormone that stabilizes our mood, feelings of well-being, and happiness. It also regulates sleep, eating and digestion.

SOY: It is a protein found in soybeans which is often used to replace animal proteins.

<u>Vitamin D3</u>: A hormone that optimizes the absorption of calcium, phosphate, and magnesium which are essential to healthy bones.

Vitamins

VITAMIN A

Anti oxidant, growth and tissue repair, sight, healthy bones and teeth. green leafy vegetables, carrots, tomatoes, mango, apricots, spinach, red and yellow peppers, brightly colored fruit and vegetables.

VITAMIN B COMPLEX

B1 thiamine, B2 riboflavin, B3 Niacin, B6 pyridoxin, folic acid, pantothenic acid. cell growth and nervous system, energy utilization. green leafy vegetables, avocado, whole grains, nuts, mushrooms, bananas, beans, lentils, oranges, bean sprouts.

VITAMIN B12

Nervous system and red cell production. Deficiency can lead to anemia and neuropathy. Should take as supplement to diet if 100% plant-based. 2500 mcg weekly recommended. Fortified products such as cereals, soy.

VITAMIN C

Anti oxidant, immune system health, wound healing. Green leafy vegetables, citrus, parsley, potatoes, broccoli, cabbage

VITAMIN D

For healthy bones and teeth. Sunshine vitamin. Fortified cereals, soy. Vitamin D3 supplement recommended 2000 IU daily.

VITAMIN E

Anti oxidant, skin, wound/tissue healing. tomatoes, apples, carrots, whole grains, nuts, seeds, avocado.

VITAMIN K

Blood clotting, healthy bones, infection fighter, energy use. green leafy vegetables, lentils, broccoli, lettuce, peas, kelp.

The B and C vitamins are considered water-soluble, meaning they will dissolve in water. Therefore, to optimize absorption of the B and C vitamins from their plant source, best to eat raw or steamed.

Minerals

All minerals come from the soil and are incorporated in plants. By eating the plants, we get all of the minerals our body needs to grow, heal and thrive. We do not need to go through a middleman such as the cow to get what we need.

CALCIUM

For healthy bones, teeth, muscles, blood clotting. Green leafy vegetables, kale, spinach, broccoli, tofu, sesame seeds.

IODINE

Essential for optimal thyroid health. Green leafy vegetables, asparagus, kelp, seaweed.

IRON

Used in production of red blood cells. 100% of daily iron requirements can easily come from a plant-based diet. Green leafy vegetables such as kale, spinach, arugula, cabbage. Beans, lentils, figs, dried apricots, dates, tofu. Vitamin C will enhance iron absorption.

MAGNESIUM

Utilized in nerve and muscle function. essential for bone strength. Whole grains, soybeans, green leafy vegetables, apples, apricots, cashews, almonds, bananas, avocados.

POTASSIUM, PHOSPHORUS, SELENIUM

Healthy bones, anti-oxidant, blood pressure. Brazil nuts, strawberries, tomatoes, bananas, chickpeas, whole grains, pumpkin seeds, many fruits, and vegetables.

TRACE ELEMENTS

Manganese, copper, cobalt, chromium, fluoride, molybdenum. Healthy bones, teeth, hair, skin, immune system. Green leafy vegetables, almonds, potatoes, bananas, seaweed, beans, lentils, whole grains.

ZINC

To maintain a strong immune system and optimize wound healing. Green leafy vegetables, almonds, tofu, whole grains, sesame and pumpkin seeds.

As you can see, eating a balanced diet of leafy green vegetables, whole grains, beans, lentils, fruits, and vegetables will cover your mineral needs. The only exception may be iodine as the iodine level in the soil where you live may vary. If there is iodine concern, then eating seaweed daily will be your best bet.

Macro-Nutrition

CARBOHYDRATES

Used for energy. Avoid simple carbohydrates such as sugars. Avoid processed grains such as white flour. Concentrate on complex carbohydrates such as beans, lentils, cereals, oats, wholegrain rice. Complex carbohydrates will represent the main source of a healthy diet.

FATS

Essential for optimal brain and nerve function. Want to get adequate omega 3 fatty acids for vascular health. Flaxseed, green leafy vegetables, avocados, nuts such as almonds, hazelnuts, cashews, walnuts represent excellent sources of healthy fat. Cooking oils are best avoided as they are not necessary and simply add excess calories. If weight not an issue then can use least amount of extra virgin olive oil. Coconut and palm oils are highly saturated and should be avoided in cooking.

FIBER

100% of fiber comes from plants and represents the residue left in the bowel post-digestion. Leads to a healthy colon with tight junctions between cells. Feeds the gut microbiome and creates an anti-inflammatory environment. Lowers cholesterol. 30 grams per day recommended. Fiber needs adequate water for optimal health, and a minimum of 2 liters per day is recommended.

PROTEIN

Essential for cell growth and repair. 30-40 grams of plant-based protein per day is all that the body needs. Plants such as spinach, kale, and broccoli contain nearly twice as much protein per weight than the leanest animal product. Undeniable worldwide data links diets with excess animal-based protein to shorter life spans.

About the Author

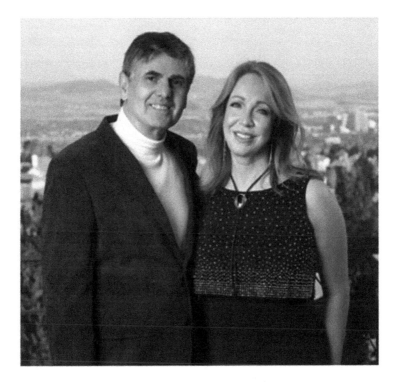

Dr. Harry and Mary Matossian

Mary Kay Matossian is a health educator and speaker. She has a B.S.N. in Nursing from the University of San Francisco, and a B.A. in Economics from Temple University in Philadelphia. She is fascinated with the observational science that supports a life free from inflammation, chronic disease, and weight gain that cause needless emotional suffering. Her biggest obsession is what factors trigger a person to believe the science to create a permanent food change for a happier, healthier body and mind.

After years of suffering from metabolic syndrome — high blood pressure, high cholesterol, high blood glucose, and a fatty liver with weight gain — she accidentally discovered how food impacts health. Her despair and confusion turned into an academic odyssey to better understand this disorder. Mary Kay Matossian is certified in the following courses: The Starch Solution by Dr. John McDougall, Whole Nutrition by Dr. Colin Campbell, AADE – American Association of Diabetes Educators. She is also a Food for Life Instructor for the Physician's Committee of Responsible Medicine. In addition, Mary is a certified yoga and meditation instructor through the Expanding Light, in Nevada City, California. Mary formulated an experiential class called,

"Truth in Food, Your Blood Knows!"

Mary has been in the healthcare industry for 25 years, working in a surgery center and endoscopy center; and she is a biometrics nurse for large corporations in Northern California.

Mary has made it her life's mission to share this simple knowledge with people to help reduce needless suffering and premature death.

Dr. Harry Matossian is a board-certified gastroenterologist. He graduated from Penn State University Medical School, and completed his medical residency at Georgetown University. He completed a gastroenterology fellowship at the University of Maryland. Dr. Matossian has seen more than 50,000 patients and ran the most cost-effective endoscopy center in Northern California, based in Lake and Mendocino counties. For more than 30 years, he has provided exemplary patient care.

Dr. Matossian continues to provide excellent medical care with the addition of introducing a whole-food, plant-based diet to his patients. Escaping the Santa Rosa fires of 2017, Mary and her husband are thriving in Reno, Nevada. Together, it is their life's mission to educate and heal people.